T0264001

Burn Care Update

Guest Editor

PATRICIA A. FORTNER, RN, MSN, MEd, CNOR, LTC

PERIOPERATIVE NURSING CLINICS

www.periopnursing.theclinics.com

Consulting Editor
NANCY GIRARD, PhD, RN, FAAN

March 2012 • Volume 7 • Number 1

SAUNDERS an imprint of ELSEVIER, Inc.

W.B. SAUNDERS COMPANY

A Division of Elsevier Inc.

1600 John F. Kennedy Boulevard • Suite 1800 • Philadelphia, Pennsylvania 19103-2899

http://www.periopnursing.theclinics.com

PERIOPERATIVE NURSING CLINICS Volume 7, Number 1
March 2012 ISSN 1556-7931, ISBN-13: 978-1-4557-3913-4

Editor: Katie Hartner
Developmental Editor: Donald Mumford

Perioperative Nursing Clinics (ISSN 1556-7931) is published quarterly by Elsevier, 360 Park Avenue South, New York, NY 10010. Months of issue are March, June, September and December. Business and Editorial Offices: 1600 John F. Kennedy Blvd., Suite 1800, Philadelphia, PA 19103-2899. Customer Service Office: 11830 Westline Industrial Drive, St. Louis, MO 63146. Periodicals postage paid at New York, NY and at additional mailing offices. Subscription prices are $132.00 per year (domestic individuals), $224.00 per year (domestic institutions), $65.00.00 per year (domestic students/ residents), $171.00 per year (international individuals), $257.00 per year (international institutions), and $69.00 per year (International students/residents). Foreign air speed delivery is included in all *Clinics* subscription prices. All prices are subject to change without notice. **POSTMASTER:** Send change of address to *Perioperative Nursing Clinics,* Customer Service (orders, claims, online, change of address): Elsevier Periodicals Customer Service, 11830 Westline Industrial Drive, St. Louis, MO 63146. Tel: 1-800-654-2452 (U.S. and Canada). Fax: 314-523-5170. E-mail: journalscustomerservice-usa@elsevier.com (for print support); journalsonlinesupport-usa@elsevier.com (for online support).

Reprints. For copies of 100 or more, of articles in this publication, please contact the Commercial Rights Department, Elsevier Inc., 360 Park Avenue South, New York, NY 10010-1710; Phone: (+1) 212-633-3813; Fax: (+1) 212-462-1935; E-mail: reprints@elsevier.com.

Printed and bound by CPI Group (UK) Ltd, Croydon, CR0 4YY
Transferred to Digital Print 2012

Contributors

CONSULTING EDITOR

NANCY GIRARD, PhD, RN, FAAN
Nurse Collaborations, Boerne, Texas; Clinical Associate Professor, Acute Nursing Care
Department, University of Texas Health Science Center, San Antonio, Texas

GUEST EDITOR

PATRICIA A. FORTNER, RN, MSN, MED, CNOR, LTC
United States Army Nurse Corps, CR Darnall Army Medical Center, Fort Hood, Texas

AUTHORS

DAVID ALLEN, MSN, RN, CCRN, CCNS-BC
Department of Behavioral Health, United States Army Institute of Surgical Research,
Fort Sam Houston, Texas

MAJ ANISSA J. BUCKLEY, RN, MSN, CNOR, ACNS
Chief, Perioperative Services, McDonald Army Health Center, Newport News, Virginia

LEOPOLDO C. CANCIO, MD, FACS
Colonel, Medical Corps, United States Army, United States Army Institute of Surgical
Research, Fort Sam Houston, Texas

RODNEY K. CHAN, MD
Division of Plastic and Reconstructive Surgery, Burn Scar Program, Dental and Trauma
Research Detachment, Burn Center, United States Army Institute of Surgical Research,
Brooke Army Medical Center, Fort Sam Houston, Texas

PETER A. DESOCIO, DO
Department of Anesthesia, The Ohio State University Medical Center, Columbus, Ohio

LTC VERNELL FLOOD, RN, MSN, PMHCNS-BC
Department of Behavioral Health, United States Army Institute of Surgical Research,
Fort Sam Houston, Texas

PATRICIA A. FORTNER, RN, MSN, MED, CNOR, LTC
United States Army Nurse Corps, CR Darnall Army Medical Center, Fort Hood, Texas

JACOB J. HANSEN, DO
United States Army Burn Center, United States Army Institute of Surgical Research,
Fort Sam Houston, Texas

BONNIE A. JACKSON, RN, MSN, CCNS-C
United States Army Institute of Surgical Research Burn Program Manager/Process
Improvement, United States Army Institute of Surgical Research-Battlefield Medicine,
Fort Sam Houston, Texas

MAJ CHRISTOPHER V. MAANI, MD, MC, US Army
Department of Anesthesiology, United States Army Institute of Surgical Research and Army Burn Center, Brooke Army Medical Center, Fort Sam Houston, Texas

DAVIN MELLUS, DMD
Division of Oral and Maxillofacial Surgery, Dental and Trauma Research Detachment, United States Army Institute of Surgical Research, Fort Sam Houston, Texas

CHRISTINA L. MOORE, CPT, AN, BSN
Burn Center, United States Army Institute of Surgical Research, San Antonio Military Medical Center, Fort Sam Houston, Texas

THERESA J. NOWAK, CPT, RN, BSN, CCRN
United States Army Institute of Surgical Research, San Antonio, Texas

PATRICIA M. SCHMIDT, CPT, AN, BSN, MHS
Burn Center, United States Army Institute of Surgical Research, San Antonio Military Medical Center, Fort Sam Houston, Texas

SARAH K. SHINGLETON, MS, RN, CCRN, CCNS
Wound Care Clinical Nurse Specialist, United States Army Institute of Surgical Research, Fort Sam Houston, Texas

MARY SUELTENFUSS, RN, BSN, NLC
Clinical Research Nurse-Pain Task Area Contractor, Cherokee Nation Technical Services (CNTS), United States Army Institute of Surgical Research-Battlefield Medicine, Fort Sam Houston, Texas

ANDREW WALLACE JR, RN, ASN
United States Army Institute of Surgical Research, Fort Sam, Houston, Texas

Contents

Preface: Burn Care Update   xi

Patricia A. Fortner

Review of Burn Treatment: Early Care to Current Practices   1

Patricia A. Fortner

> Management and care of the burn patient has advanced since early
> times and will continue to advance. The author traces burns past and
> present; reviews history and advances in grafting, skin substitutes and
> dressings; and discusses tools and treatments.

Burn Pathophysiology   9

Theresa J. Nowak

> Treating burns is complex because the body undergoes a myriad of
> changes that affect every system. The likelihood of survival diminishes
> with advanced age, existence of comorbidities, and extent of body
> surface area and inhalation injury. The stress response and burn shock
> are the two chief physiologic processes that overwhelm the victim
> initially and following burn injury. Inflammatory mediators consume the
> body, altering normal function of all organs. These alterations will have
> life-threatening consequences if misdiagnosed. Providers must be
> properly trained in the recognition of all aspects of burn care to allow
> their patients the greatest chance of survival.

Caring for the Burn Patient: The Perioperative Nurse   19

Bonnie A. Jackson and Mary Sueltenfuss

> This article discusses the role and responsibilities of the perioperative
> nurse in burn care and describes phases of care during treatment and
> recovery and the respect and compassion needed in caring for the burn
> patient.

Perioperative Anesthetic Considerations for Burn Patients   23

Christopher V. Maani, Jacob J. Hansen, Patricia A. Fortner,
Leopoldo C. Cancio, and Peter A. DeSocio

> Military health care providers face the challenge of treating severely burned
> soldiers and civilians. Burn patients have perioperative anesthesia con-
> cerns distinct from other surgical populations. These issues require con-
> sideration and planning by the surgical team and the anesthesia provider.
> The authors discuss anesthetic and perioperative considerations for these
> patients that may be encountered by perioperative nurses, based on their

experience at the US Army Institute of Surgical Research Burn Center at Brooke Army Medical Center, Fort Sam Houston, Texas. With proper planning and close coordination with the burn care team, burn patients can be cared for effectively, compassionately, and safely.

Perioperative Nursing Considerations in Burn Care   35

Patricia A. Fortner

Patients with severe burns require specialized care because of their susceptibility to infection and potential complications from inhalation injury and/or shock. Certain wound treatments and specialized operative interventions have been shown to reduce patient length of stay. These treatments, including skin grafting surgeries and highly specialized wound care, are best delivered in burn centers and are important in increasing the likelihood of survival and reducing complications and adverse outcomes. This article describes causes and types of burns, hypothermia concerns, operating room conditions and preparation, surgical intervention, types of skin substitutions, and the special demands on perioperative burn nurses.

Surgical Care of Thermally Injured Patients on the Battlefield   53

Leopoldo C. Cancio

For young adults treated in burn centers in developed nations, burn size lethal to one-half of the population has almost doubled since World War II, from 43% to 75% of the total body surface area. This achievement reflects improvements in wound care, perioperative care, and surgical technique. The current challenge military health care providers face is how to translate these advances to the combat zone. The author discusses surgical care of patients with thermal injuries as currently practiced on the battlefield and during resuscitation, wound closure, and reconstruction phases.

A Burn Intensive Care Unit Nurse's Perspective   71

Andrew Wallace Jr

Burn care requires constant communication and attention to detail, as well as mental and physical toughness. From the warm environment and long hours at the bedside caring for the patient to the interaction with the families, burn nurses are at the front of patient care. The author discusses aspects of burn care including characteristics of burns, patient transport and specialized operating room procedures, medications and fluids, and postoperative concerns.

Hope for Recovering Burn Patients—The Multidisciplinary Approach (Ultrarapid Opioid Detoxification Under Anesthesia)   77

Bonnie A. Jackson, Mary Sueltenfuss, and Christopher V. Maani

Burn patients must endure countless wound debridement procedures, dressing changes, and multiple surgeries, and acute pain can become unrelenting chronic pain. Currently, medications that act on μ-opioid receptors have proven to provide the best pharmacologic management for the relief of chronic burn-related pain. As a result, opioid analgesia has risen to the forefront of the health care professional's arsenal for the treatment of burn pain. However, prolonged opioid therapy can leave a recovering burn patient with opioid dependence or addiction. This article discusses multidisciplinary ultrarapid detoxification under anesthesia, including protocols, patient evaluation, staffing, procedures, and lessons learned.

Battlefield Pain Control: Forging Ahead by Building on the Past   83

Christopher V. Maani

Reduction of unnecessary pain and suffering is a cornerstone of medicine. Along with the mental anguish of being in pain, there are long-term sequelae, which may include posttraumatic stress disorder, depression, nonrestorative sleep patterns, and chronic pain syndromes. Solving the problem of excessive pain may prove more challenging in military than civilian populations. Tactical considerations of austere and far-forward care such as noise and light discipline, as well as the ability to maintain an effective fighting force, complicate the care of combat casualties. This article addresses battlefield pain options currently available as well as analgesic alternatives being developed.

Pressure Ulcers in the Burned Patient: Perioperative Considerations   89

Sarah K. Shingleton

All surgical patients should be considered at risk for developing pressure ulcers. Burn patients are especially at risk for further skin and tissue injury. Key components of a perioperative pressure injury prevention strategy include thorough skin assessments, interventions to reduce shear and friction during patient positioning and transfer, and use of pressure redistribution surfaces and overlays. A collaborative approach involving the multidisciplinary burn team is vital in the ongoing care of the burned patient and is essential to the achievement of positive outcomes and maintenance of a safe patient environment.

A Burn Progressive Care Unit: Customized Care from Admission Through Discharge   99

Christina L. Moore and Patricia M. Schmidt

Caring for burn patients forms special bonds between burn center staff, patients, and the patients' families. This connection begins on admission and continues throughout the healing process, which may last for years. The authors, Army nurses, describe nursing care in a progressive burn unit starting with patient admission from intensive burn care to this lower-acuity phase and including transferring to the unit, standard routines, nutrition, surgery, postoperative care, and discharge from the unit.

Reconstructive Surgery in the Thermally Injured Patient   107

Davin Mellus and Rodney K. Chan

Although the operations required during acute burn hospitalization are life saving, subsequent reconstructive operations can be life giving. Each reconstructive plan is tailored for each patient, depending on the specific deformity. Multiple reconstructive modalities are possible, but the goal is always restoration of form and function. The operative plan must include preoperative, intraoperative, and postoperative considerations to be successful.

Trauma-Induced Coagulopathy: An Update to Current Management   115

Christopher V. Maani and Peter A. DeSocio

Trauma-induced coagulopathy and bleeding after severe injury represent a problem that is challenging to manage and even more difficult to reverse. When caring for patients showing signs of hemorrhagic shock, clinicians must anticipate, recognize, and manage the coagulopathy of trauma as close to the onset of injury as possible. The longer left untreated, the greater likelihood that a patient will develop hemorrhagic shock and multiorgan system failure. Uncompensated hemorrhage often predisposes trauma patients to higher mortality rates, highlighting the need for recognizing and treating the main influences in coagulopathy of trauma with the newest evidence-based practices.

High-Tech, High-Stress Environment: Coping Strategies for the Perioperative Nurse   129

Vernell Flood and David Allen

The operating room (OR) is among the most technologically advanced environments within the healthcare profession. This environment has a unique set of occupational demands that can cause increased stress for the nursing staff. Situations that lead nurses to experience pressure in the OR include the need to work quickly, face higher medical dispute risks, work uncertain shifts, handle precision instruments, and master complex techniques. Along with this, perioperative nurses struggle with heavy workloads, high patient acuity, various instrument processing issues, low morale, and staff shortages. The nurse must skillfully manage these tasks while keeping patient safety at the forefront.

Behind the Redline: Personal Experiences of a Perioperative Burn Nurse in the Military   135

Anissa J. Buckley

> A perioperative nurse describes firsthand experiences during an assignment in the burn center at the US Army Institute of Surgical Research. Unique aspects and demands of the burn unit versus typical perioperative care are depicted, along with portrayals of two memorable patients.

Index   139

FORTHCOMING ISSUES

June 2012

Informatics
Joy Don Baker, PhD, RN-BC, CNE, CNOR, NEA-BC, *Guest Editor*

September 2012

Change Strategies
Mickey L. Parsons, PhD, MHA, RN, FAAN, *Guest Editor*

December 2012

Nurse Advocacy
Terri Goodman, PhD, RN, *Guest Editor*

RECENT ISSUES

December 2011

Collaborative Care of the Facial Injury Patient
Vivek Shetty, DDS, Dr Med Dent, and Grant N. Marshall, PhD, *Guest Editors*

September 2011

Robotic Surgery
John Zender, RN, BS, CNOR, *Guest Editor*

June 2011

Plastic and Reconstructive Surgery
Deborah S. Hickman Mathis, RN, MS, CNOR, RNFA, *Guest Editor*

Preface
Burn Care Update

Since the beginning of time, fire has been man's friend and foe and has helped and harmed him. Fire provided man with the tools to advance humankind, but also jumped out at him and caused him immeasurable pain and grief.

The challenges presented by a thermal injury are numerous. Burns have always left an indelible impression on the victims, their families, and their caregivers because they often lead to protracted suffering with fatal consequences, or to disfiguring scars, functional disorders, or social isolation. Morbidity and mortality statistics have improved with the development of specialty burn centers, fellowship-trained burn physicians, and dedicated multidisciplinary burn teams. Burn experts provide surgical and critical care, psychiatric services, respiratory therapy, clinical nutrition, physical and occupational therapy, case management and social work services, infection prevention, chaplain, and outpatient services. Specially trained burn nurses provide perioperative, critical, transitional, wound, psychiatric, and outpatient care. Burn care teams are knowledgeable, flexible, and dedicated. No one team member stands alone; each is prepared with compassion and empathy to care for the burn victim to the best of their ability.

Current burn care evolved from the practices of the forefathers of today's burn surgeons. And while surgeons of the 21st century no longer use fat from very old wild hogs or graft frog skin on burns to treat their patients, modern science has developed new technologies that are based on old practices. In this issue of *Perioperative Nursing Clinics*, Fortner reviews the care and treatment of burns in antiquity and the development of modern remedies, all tried and trialed on burn patients of the past.

Nowak explains the zones of a burn injury, factors determining the severity of a burn wound, and the classification of burns, all critical knowledge that a provider must possess in order to treat the burn victim properly. Her article describes the pathophysiology of burns: the stress response and burn shock that patients experience after burn injuries. Jackson and Sueltenfuss wrote an outstanding article on Watson's Caring theory as it applies to the perioperative phases in a burn operating room. They explain how perioperative nurses (as do all burn nurses and doctors) become the strength of the patient because of the caring that each has within them for their patients.

Perioperative Anesthetic Considerations for Burn Patients by Maani and colleagues is a comprehensive discussion of the unique anesthesia concerns of the burn patient. Preoperative considerations are noted and induction of anesthesia, blood loss, and drugs used intraoperatively are discussed. In Perioperative Considerations for the Burn Patient, Fortner discusses criteria for admission to a burn center, common causes of burns, determination of the severity of burns, mortality in burn injuries, and initial treatment of the patient. Preparation in the operating room for surgical intervention, perioperative teamwork involving the nursing staff, anesthesia, and the surgeon and the conduction of the surgical procedure are discussed.

Perioperative Nursing Clinics 7 (2012) xi–xiii
doi:10.1016/j.cpen.2012.01.001
1556-7931/12/$ – see front matter © 2012 Elsevier Inc. All rights reserved.

periopnursing.theclinics.com

Equipment, instruments, supplies, surgical procedures, dressings, and skin substitutes are noted.

Cancio describes the three phases of burn care, initial burn management, and topical agents used and details surgical intervention in a burn center and a deployed setting. Before and after surgery, the Burn Intensive Care Unit cares for the major burn patient. Wallace describes the role of the nurse, drugs used postoperatively, and the care of different grafts and donor sites. Along with treating the burn wound, specially trained burn teams must also consider the patient's pain. Patients who sustain major burns are subjected to multiple debridements, dressing changes, and countless surgical procedures and may develop a physical dependence or addiction to narcotics. Jackson and coworkers' article on Ultra Rapid Opioid Detoxification under Anesthesia is a fascinating look at anesthesia's process of minimizing opioid use and managing the patient's pain while avoiding debilitating withdrawal symptoms.

Battlefield Pain Control by Maani discusses pain management processes used currently in hospitals and burn centers and elaborates on strategies used in far-forward deployed combat situations. Burn pain (considered to be the worst possible pain) has been shown to respond to immersive virtual reality (iVR). Maani explains how iVR can be used to provide analgesia for a burn patient, which could result in minimizing sedation, maximizing pain control, and helping our wounded warriors and all burn patients tolerate painful dressing changes, minor procedures, and evacuation from a war zone.

Pressure Ulcers in the Burned Patient written by Shingleton reviews the complications of pressure ulcers in the non-burned patient and goes on to note the relationship between pressure ulcer formation and the pathophysiology of the burn patient. Comorbidities and factors that place the burn patient at increased risk of developing a pressure ulcer are written about in depth.

Assessment and risk determination, intraoperative considerations, critical care unit considerations, and preventive recommendations are addressed. An article written by Moore and Schmidt walks the reader through a progressive care unit and describes goals of the unit, the daily care of the burn patient, and the teamwork that leads a patient to discharge. The nursing care for the patient on this step down unit is explained and includes fluid and electrolyte balance, pain control, medications, hydrotherapy, dressings, rehabilitation, and preparing the patient for discharge.

After the initial burn injury and subsequent surgical procedures, patients often require reconstructive surgery. Mellus and Chan describe the role of the reconstructive surgeon for burn patients and the procedures that assist the burn patient in their recovery. Reconstructive Surgery in the Thermally Injured Patient details diagnosis and appraisal, goals of the surgical intervention, and perioperative considerations.

Maani and DeSocio review the literature concerning trauma-induced coagulopathy. In their article, they discuss the perspective of hemorrhage as it pertains to the trauma patient, and the concept of damage control resuscitation currently used in far-forward combat settings. An in-depth explanation of the factors that affect coagulopathy and the resuscitation and management of the condition is noted.

Flood and Allen discuss the high-stress environment of the perioperative arena and the increase of occupational stress all burn nurses endure as they care for this challenging patient population. High-Tech, High-Stress Environment: Coping Skills for the Perioperative Nurse details strategies that all health care providers can use in stressful workplaces. Last, Buckley discusses her personal experiences in Behind the Red Line: Personal Experiences of a Perioperative Burn Nurse in the Military.

The articles contained in this issue of *Perioperative Nursing Clinics* demonstrate the underlying commonality of burn patient caregivers. The multidisciplinary, multiskilled, focused burn team works together to provide extraordinary care to this unique population. The successful management of the burn patient is a long, difficult journey but the community of clinicians who care for these patients has a depth of knowledge, experience, and commitment that is unrivaled.

My sincere appreciation to all of the authors who wrote about their work and to the editors at Elsevier who worked tirelessly to bring this issue to publication. Thank you.

Patricia A. Fortner, RN, MSN, MEd, CNOR
United States Army Nurse Corps
CR Darnall Army Medical Center
Fort Hood, TX 76544, USA

E-mail address:
pat.fortner@us.army.mil

Review of Burn Treatment: Early Care to Current Practices

Patricia A. Fortner, RN, MSN, MEd, CNOR

KEYWORDS
- Burn treatment • Nursing care • History • Current practices

FIRE

In Greek mythology, the Titian Prometheus who was also known as Forethought, traveled to live among men and help them. He grew very sad when he saw that man was poor and wretched and dwelled in caves, was cold because there was no fire, was starving and was hunted by other men and the wild animals that roamed the earth. Prometheus discovered that man was the most miserable of creatures.

Prometheus asked the god Jupiter to give man fire so he could survive the coming winter, but Jupiter refused saying that if men had fire, they would become strong like the gods. Jupiter said that man should remain poor, and ignorant, living like beasts so that the gods could continue to be all mighty and all powerful.

Prometheus, as Forethought, looked toward the future and knew that he must give mortal man the gift of fire. He touched a fennel stalk to a ray of the sun and it began to burn. Prometheus stole carefully to the land of man and called the men from their caves and showed them how to build a fire and how to build other fires from the coals. Men and their women soon learned how to cook their food and eat like men and not like the beasts that had hunted them. They came out of the dark places in which they had previously dwelled and were happy. According to Greek mythology, a new and golden age had begun.

The beginning of the use of fire is unknown; its origin can only be guessed at. The Paleolithic Man placed drawings of fire on the walls of the caves that he lived in. How man came to possess this special discovery will never be determined. Did he transfer hot lava from a nearby volcano or take a burning branch off of a tree that had been struck by lightning? Or did he make that first fire by rubbing two sticks together?

However man found fire, we also wonder how he developed its use. How did he decide to mix clay with water and bake it into vessels for liquids and for cooking use?

The opinions or assertions contained herein are the private views of the author and are not to be construed as official or as reflecting the views of the Department of the Army or the Department of Defense.

United States Army Nurse Corps, CR Darnall Army Medical Center, Fort Hood, TX 76544, USA

E-mail address: pat.fortner@us.army.mil

How did man discover that he could bend metal into implements and weapons? However this occurred, fire played an important part in the progression of man during prehistoric times.

While fire played a significant role in the development of modern man, fire also had the ability to harm him. The consequences of burns to man resulted in a plethora of treatments, salves, and potions.

BURN TREATMENT

The first known writings concerning the treatment of burn wounds seem to be the Eber Papyrus, around 1500 BC. Applications of black mud, yeasty dough made with cow dung, cereal made of barley, a mixture of mashed beans and beeswax, and creams made with red ochre and copper were described. Other treatments consisted of ram's hair mixed with the milk of a woman who had recently given birth to a male child and boiled goat excrement, herbs, and onions applied while a healer chanted, "Water is in my mouth, a Nile is between my thighs. I have come to extinguish the fire."[1]

Throughout history a number of famous philosophers, physicians, and scientists have contributed to the knowledge of burn management, including such notables as Hippocrates, Celsus, Pliny the Elder, Galen, Aristotle, Rhases, Clowes, Pare, Hildanus, Marjolin, Dupuytren, and Syme.[2] These men contributed to the treatment of burn wounds with the use of various plants, gums, tea leaves, roasted angleworms, oak bark extract, honey, cork, bear fat, bran, ashes, vinegar, wine, fat from "very old wild hogs," calcium chloride soaks, moss "from the skull of a person hung," red sandalwood, cold water, saline baths, lemon strips soaked in oily dressings, soot, spiderwebs, linseed oil mixed with lime water, picric acid, medicated paraffin, carbolic acid, cod liver oil, and portions "of a genuine mummy."[3–6]

GRAFTS

The Brahmin Koomes Caste reported that Susrata, from a bricklaying class of people, performed the first plastic surgery when he grafted new noses from skin flaps in India in 800 BC. Amputating the nose was considered punishment for theft and adultery; the likely donors were unwilling slaves.[6,7] (According to Ang,[8] amputation of the nose was practiced until at least 1983 in Afghanistan and Pakistan).

Hildanus, a 15th century German physician, was the first to classify burns into three degrees.[9] Hildanus classified them on the basis of their appearance and described the most superficial burns as red and blistered, deeper burns as withering but not charring the skin, and the deepest as those with eschar and charred skin.[10] Hildanus also advocated that for deep burns, incisions should be made "to let the moisture escape."[11]

Tagliacozzi successfully transplanted skin flaps from the patients' own arms to recreate their noses in the 16th century. In 1682, Canady reported on the use of lizard skin for wound closure, and since then, the membranous lining of eggs; the skins of chickens, guinea pigs, rabbits, and pigs; and amniotic membranes have been used in the treatment of burn wounds.[10] About 1700, human skin is believed to have been transplanted to burn, disease, and injury patients in India. The first burn hospital was not created until 1843, when a cottage on the grounds of the Edinburgh Royal Infirmary was dedicated to men and women with severe burns. Later it was discovered that this part of the hospital was established only because "the surgeons . . . wanted these damned stinking things out of their wards."[12]

Reverdin, a Swiss physician, is credited with describing the first fresh allograft (now considered the gold standard in biological dressings) in 1869, although earlier attempts at skin transplantation by other surgeons are mentioned in literature, including Cooper in 1817 and Buenger in 1821.[13] Reverdin later perfected the pinch graft, which removed tiny sections of healthy skin and transplanted them to areas that needed to be covered.

Ollier, in Paris or Lyons, France, reported on and coined the term *dermoepidermic grafting* in 1871.[14] Ollier emphasized the importance of the dermal and epidermal transplantation throughout the literature in 1872.[12,15,16] Girdner also claimed to perform the first allografts in 1881.[16] Some investigators also give credit to Pollock of London, who published a series of articles dealing with the subject in 1870[12] and is reported to have performed the first free flap on a burn wound.

Early surgeons continued to cover open burn wounds with all sorts of substances (frog, chicken, or rabbit skin, and so forth), autograft (tissue transferred from one part of the body to another), allograft (tissue transferred from a genetically different individual of the same species: cadaver skin), and xenograft (tissue transferred from an individual of another species: porcine/pig skin). Autograft has been the most successful. Allograft is considered a temporary, biological wound covering. Xenograft is considered a manufactured biological dressing.

TREATMENT OF BURN WOUNDS

Early burn treatment described sealing of the burn wound. Although this method decreased the patient's pain and was thought to decrease the incidence of blister formation, it in fact allowed bacteria to thrive and multiply, and burn victims subsequently died a tortured death.

World War I produced few new burn therapies. Most burns were treated as they had been a hundred years before. Bicarbonate of soda dressings or saline solutions were used to cleanse the wound and soothe the pain. Morphine was used for severe cases.[17] Picric acid (also used in bomb-making in World War I) was used by surgeons. Picric acid is a coagulating agent that formed a membrane over the wound. It did ease pain, but it so firmly stuck to the dressings that when they were removed, healing tissue was removed as well.

The French advocated the use of a 96% paraffin treatment. The paraffin was liberally sprayed on and protected the burn from painful air flow. It did seal in toxins, but as the patient moved, the seal broke and plasma drained from the wound. Dichloramin-T a form of Carrel-Dakin solution was used as a neutralizing agent against mustard gas burns in 1917.[17]

Later, in 1925, physicians began to use tannic acid for burn wounds, although tannic acid treatment had been practiced for 5000 years by folk healers who soaked leaves in a dilute solution of tannic acid. Davidson at Henry Ford Hospital in Detroit performed sterile debridements of burn blisters and then sprayed the wound with a 5% aqueous solution of tannic acid every 15 minutes until a dark mahogany-colored coagulum was obtained. This usually required from 10 to 18 hours.[18] In 1943, McClure reported that tannic acid was toxic to the liver, and its use was discontinued.[19] In 1933, Aldrich began using gentian violet after debridement of burn wounds and later prescribed a triple combination dye (gentian violet, brilliant green, and yellow acriflavine) after debridement.

The first true description of excisional therapy for deep burns was likely described by Lustgarten in 1891 and performed by Wilms in 1901.[11] Early excisional therapy of the burn wound with subsequent grafting gained increased attention with the 1942 publication by Cope and colleagues.[19] Cope had cared for burn patients from the infamous Coconut Grove Nightclub fire and noted that patients undergoing excisional debridement of their wounds did better than those that did not. In the early 1950s, spurred on by thermal injuries during the Korean War, the US government established the original Surgical Research Unit (The United States Army Burn Center) at Brooke Army Hospital in San Antonio, Texas, where skin grafting became the preferred treatment for 30% total body surface area burns.[9] Several reports are scattered throughout the literature over the next 30 years,[20] but reports were discouraging because they showed little clinical improvement over the usual practice of waiting for spontaneous eschar separation followed by grafting on granulation tissue.[21] In 1970, Janzekovic described tangential excision of burns. This method involved the surgical removal of successive layers of the dead skin down to viable dermis. When living tissue was reached, it was covered with a skin graft. Janzekovic solidified the concept of early excision and grafting in the burn community.[14] The efficacy of this technique was confirmed in groundbreaking study by Heimbach.[17] This seminal study confirmed that early excision of burns lowered costs, shortened hospital stays, and lowered burn mortality—a goal that has been sought since burn care was undertaken.[22]

TOOLS (OF THE TRADE)

Advancements in the technical aspects of skin grafting continued slowly. Initial grafts were obtained free-handed with long, thin-bladed knives.[23] In 1886, Thiersch, a German surgeon, developed a method using a straight razor that excised long strips of split skin graft that used the epidermis and a portion of the dermis and applied them to freshly debrided granulation tissue bed.[14,15,24] In 1920, Finochietto developed a calibrated knife, a primitive mechanical skin harvesting device to excise wounds. In 1929, Blair and Brown developed improved techniques of split-thickness skin grafting, which allowed the use of varying dermal thicknesses and resulted in less shrinkage and contracture of the burn wound. Blair later developed another such skin grafting knife combined with a suction apparatus for removing the graft. Braithwaite, Watson, Goulian, and Corbett are names still associated with knives used to harvest skin and remove burned tissues.[14]

In the years to follow, various attempts were made to develop a mechanical device to facilitate the harvesting of skin grafts. One of the greatest advances in skin grafting was the development of the dermatome. The first device was invented by Humbly of England and was introduced in the 1930s. The introduction 9 years later of the hand-powered rotating drum dermatome by Padgett, a surgeon, and Hood, a mechanical engineer, was also a significant advancement because it provided quick, accurate, and uniform split-thickness skin grafts. The first powered dermatome was invented by Brown.[24] According to several authors, Brown conceived of the instrument while being held prisoner by the Japanese during World War II.[12] Introduced in 1948, it revolutionized the treatment of open wounds and burns and remains one of the most important tools of the burn surgeon.

Lanz constructed a primitive mesher in 1908. In the early 1960s Tanner and Vandeput developed a hand-cranked double roller meshing device that permitted up to a nine-fold expansion of split-thickness skin grafts and reduced the need for reharvesting of the few available donor sites on patients with extensive burns.[10,18] The mesher is also considered a vital part of the burn surgeon's toolbox.

TOPICAL ANTIMICROBIAL AGENTS

Effective topical antimicrobial agents decrease infection, drastically reduce mortality in burn patients, and play an important role in the management of burn patients today. Dakin solution was first developed in 1915 by Dakin, who was investigating a number of antiseptic substances including phenol, salicylic acid, hydrogen peroxide, iodine, mercuric chloride, and sodium hypochlorite. Dakin concluded that hypochlorite had a high germicidal action but that commercial products available and derived from Berthollet's 1788 solution of sodium chloride and sodium hypochlorite were far too irritating and caustic for general use.

Dakin described a method of hypochlorite synthesis devoid of irritating contaminants that produced an end concentration of 0.5% to 0.6% sodium hypochlorite. This solution could be continuously applied to wounds for more than a week without irritation.[25] Dakin solution was used in World War II for burns but was largely discontinued with the introduction of antibiotics. It was reintroduced in the 1980s[26] and is used in the treatment of gram-positive and gram-negative bacteria in burn patients.

One percent silver sulfadiazine (Silvadene) has been a traditional method of burn care for more than 30 years. It is a water-soluble cream that contains silver nitrate and silver sulfadiazine. Silvadene is used to decrease bacterial colonization of burn wounds and to treat a broad spectrum of pathogens. Unlike silver nitrate it does not stain, and unlike mafenide it is not painful for the patient. Silver sulfadiazine 1% was introduced n the mid-1960s.

Mafenide acetate (Sulfamylon) is an antimicrobial agent that exerts broad bacteriostatic action against many gram-negative and gram-positive organisms including Pseudomonas. It was first introduced as mafenide hydrochloride in 1938 as an oral antibiotic, but it proved to be ineffective. In World War II, German physicians found that mafenide was effective for wounds with blood and pus. In 1943, the British captured supplies of mafenide. The United States later obtained possession of the captured mafenide, and it was stored for years in Maryland. In 1950, Mendelson found that a topical 10% solution or a 20% aqueous of mafenide solution increased the survival rate of goats with blast injuries and that mafenide possessed Pseudomonas-resistant properties. The Army Burn Center affirmed mafenide's efficacy against Pseudomonas in human trials beginning in 1964, resulting in a decrease in burn-associated deaths. Mafenide is available as a 5% powder and a 10% cream and is an important tool in the burn surgeon's arsenal because it penetrates eschar and is effective against invading bacteria.

The antimicrobial properties of silver nitrate and its compounds have been used in medicine since the early 19th century. Halstead of Johns Hopkins Hospital wrapped wounds in silver foil and used silver suture in 1895. Five percent and 10% silver nitrate solutions were used in both world wars for burns but were largely abandoned at the end of World War II because of the hard eschar that formed. Beginning in 1960, Moyer began using 0.5% silver nitrate on burns and grafted areas. Moyer found that silver nitrate was effective against *Staphylococcus aureus*, *Pseudomonas aeruginosa* and hemolytic streptococci without the development of resistance.[27] Fifty years after Moyer began using the diluted solution, 0.5% and 0.25% silver nitrate solutions remain in use for burn patients. Silver nitrate cannot penetrate eschar and stains anything it touches.

Bacitracin is a nontoxic water-soluble topical antibiotic used chiefly against gram-positive organisms of burn wounds but not against gram-negative organisms or fungi. It is used often on face burns.

SKIN SUBSTITUTES

There are a number of commercially available products to facilitate permanent wound coverage. Integra is a bilayer skin substitute made of bovine collagen and shark chondroitin sulfate with a silicone surface layer. It is considered a regeneration template because skin cells grow through it. It is applied to a well-vascularized wound that is free from infection. After revascularization, the silicone layer is removed and is replaced by a thin layer of split-thickness skin graft. Integra provides good aesthetic results.

AlloDerm is an acellular, derived from human cadaver, dermal-regeneration matrix devoid of epidermis. It must be sandwiched with a thin split-thickness autograft at the time of the initial surgical intervention. It was developed because acellular dermal matrices are not usually rejected. It is processed in a salt water solution and freeze-dried.

Cultured epidermal autografts (Epicel) are grown from the patient's epidermal cells in tissue cultures. A skin biopsy is taken from the patient; the dermis and subcutaneous tissue are removed in a laboratory and the epidermis is mixed with irradiated mouse fibroblasts. After several weeks of tissue culture growth in the laboratory the matured sheets of cultured keratinocytes are applied to the patient's burn wound. Each graft has a petroleum gauze backing and is approximately 50 cm in diameter. Epicel is expensive, ranging from $6000 to $10,000 per 1% total body surface area burn.

Biobrane is used as a temporary cover for clean debrided burn wounds and is a synthetic, bilaminate membrane with an outer semipermeable silicone layer coated with porcine dermal collagen. It is elastic and transparent, allowing for patient movement and easy inspection of the burn wound.

TransCyte is also a temporary skin substitute. It is combined with cryopreserved Biobrane and growth factors from neonatal foreskin. It is no longer available because of manufacturer's financial factors.

Dermagraft is a synthetic product similar to TransCyte but lacks the silicone layer.

DRESSINGS

Early care of burns involved either closed dressings or open exposure. In 1887, the Alabama surgeon Copeland[10] first proposed an open technique of burn wound treatment. In one case described in the literature, Copeland left dressings off of the burn, put the patient's burned hands in pasteboard boxes, and did not allow anything to touch the burned surfaces. The ends of the box were cut out to fit the wrists, and they were covered with mosquito netting to keep out the flies. When pus was found to be accumulating under the scab, a small opening was made at one edge and the secretions were pressed out by means of a soft, dry piece of lint.[28] This method fell out of popular use because of infection.

In 1949, Wallace of Edinburgh, Scotland, again began to use the open exposure method for the treatment of burns. After a prolonged evaluation the method was reported in 1952 with the belief that when properly applied it offered many advantages over the well-established technique of occlusive dressings.[7,29] The open method was used more readily in the southern United States because the warm climate was conducive to infection under large bulky absorptive dressings. In addition, exposure was more comfortable and permitted drying of the burned surface with decreased incidence of infection. In the northern part of the country, burns most often occur in the winter months, and patients found exposure uncomfortable on the cold wards. If blankets are applied to increase comfort, a warm, humid environment is produced, which prevents the formation of a clean, dry protective covering. It soon became evident that dressings were much more comfortable in a cold climate, and proper exposure was difficult to achieve.[7]

In 1942, Allen and Koch popularized a petrolatum gauze and dressing closure method that decreased surface drying. The primary cause of death from burns at that time was septicemia from burn infection, and many surgeons began using the exposure method after the introduction of silver sulfadiazine and Sulfamylon. Later, petroleum-impregnated gauze use was begun again and continues to be the dressing of choice for donor sites in many hospitals.

Silver nitrate soaks required an occlusive dressing and were the first use of a moist wound healing method in burns overall. However, the main concept in burn care was not wet or dry, but rather control of infection by topical antibiotics.[30]

Surface drying of the burn wound was found not only to impede delivery of nutrients and immune defenses but also to markedly impede the ability of cells to migrate across the wound surface. Epithelial cells need a moisture layer to migrate and spread. For any reepithelialization to occur on a dry surface, the cells must burrow beneath the scab using a controlled release of proteases.[30] Healing under both wet and moist environments has been clearly demonstrated to be significantly faster than under dry conditions.[31] Moist healing provides rapid movement of epithelial cells across the burned surface and decreased inflammation.

The best approach to maintaining a moist wound surface is the use of an occlusive dressing. Plastic bags have been used on burned extremities to retain the dressing's moisture. Cotton roller stretch gauze covered by elastic bandages and wetted down at close intervals is most frequently used. The type of dressing used on the burn patient is dictated by surgeon choice and local standards.

SUMMARY

The management and care of the burn patient from early times when humans were first given fire to the present have changed drastically. From animal excrement and incantations to antimicrobial agents and modern-day surgical intervention, burn care has grown and will continue to grow with the goal of helping ease the terrible burden of the burn injury. And although much has been done to prevent fires, we live in a violent world in which fires in homes, vehicles, industrial settings, wars, and nature will put people at risk for the rest of our history.[12]

REFERENCES

1. Scarborough J. On medications for burns in classical antiquity. Clin Plast Surg 1983;10:603–10.
2. Barillo DJ. Topical antimicrobials in burn wound care: a recent history. Wounds 2008;20(7):192–8.
3. Moncrief JA. The development of topical therapy. J Trauma 1971;11:906–10.
4. Tenenhaus M, Rennekampff HO. Burn surgery. Clin Plast Surg 2007;34:697–715.
5. Girdner JH. Skin grafting with graft taken from the dead subject. The Medical Record (NY) 1881;20:119–20.
6. Peterson HD. Topical antibacterials. In: Bostick JA Jr, editor. The art and science of burn care. Rockville (MD): Aspen Publishers; 1987. p. 33–55.
7. Hauben DJ, Baruchin A, Mahler A. On the history of the free skin graft. Ann Plast Surg 1982;9(3):242–5.
8. Ang GC. History of skin transplantation. Clin Dermatol 2005;23(4):320–4.
9. Weeks BS. Brief introduction to the history of burns medical science. In: Xu RX, Sun X, Weeks BS, editors. Burns regenerative medicine and therapy. New York: Karger; 2004. p. 1–3.
10. Cioffi WG, Rue WG, Buescher TM, et al. A brief history of burn care. In: Zajtchuk R, Jenkins DP, Bellamy RF, editors. Conventional warfare: ballistic, blast, and burn injuries. Washington, DC: Office of the Surgeon General, Department of the Army, Borden Institute; 1990.p. 337–48.
11. Copeland WP. The treatment of burns. The Medical Record (NY) 1887:31;518.

12. Klasen HJ. History of burns. Rotterdam (The Netherlands): Erasmus Publishing; 2004.
13. Chick LR. Brief history and biology of skin grafting. Ann Plast Surg 1988;21(4):358–65.
14. Paul CN. Skin grafting in burns. Wounds-a Compendium of Clinical Research and Practice 2008;20(7):199–202.
15. Haynes FW. The history of burn care. In: Bostwick JA, editor. The art and science of burn care. Rockville (MD): Aspen Publishers; 1987. p. 3–9.
16. Artz CP. History of burns. In: Artz CP, Moncrief JA, Pruitt BA, editors. Burns: a team approach. Philadelphia: WB Saunders; 1979. p. 3–16.
17. Heimbach DM. The results of early primary excision. J Trauma 1981;21;732–4.
18. National Research Council (U.S.), Division of Medical Sciences, Office of Medical Information. Report on the treatment of thermal burns; general outline. 1943.
19. Janzekovic Z. A New concept in the early excision and immediate grafting of burns. J Trauma 1970;19:1103–8.
20. Switzer W, Jones J, Monchrief J. Evaluation of early excision of burns in children. J Trauma 1965;5:540.
21. Heimbach DM, Faucher LD. Principles of burn surgery. In: Barret JP, Herndon DN, editors. Principles and practice of burn surgery. New York: Marcel Dekker; 2005. p. 135.
22. Feller I, Tholen D, Cornell RG. Improvements in burn care 1965 to1878. JAMA 1980;244(18):2074–8.
23. McClure RD, Allen CI. Davidson tannic acid treatment of burns: ten year results. Am J Surgery 1935;28(2):370–88.
24. Tanner JC Jr, Vandeput J, Olley JF. The mesh skin graft. Plast Reconstr Surg 1964;34:287–92.
25. Dakin HD. On the use of certain antiseptic substances in the treatment of infected wounds. Br Med J 1915;2(2852):318–20.
26. Heggers JP, Sazy JA, Stenberg BD, et al. Bacterial and wound healing properties of sodium hypochlorite solutions: the 1991 Lindberg award. J Burn Care Rehabil 1991;12(5):420–4.
27. Moyer C, Brentano L, Gravens DL, et al. Treatment of large human burns with 0.5% silver nitrate solution. Arch Surg 1965;90:81267.
28. Artz CP, Reiss E, Davis JH Jr, et al. The exposure treatment of burns.Ann Surg 1953;137:456.
29. Artz CP, Gaston BH. A reappraisal of the exposure method in the treatment of burns, donor sites and skin grafts. Ann Surg 1960;151(6):939–50.
30. Demling RH, DeSanti L, Orgill DP. Moist healing and wound care including burns. Burn Surg 2000.
31. Atiyeh BS, Hayek SN. Intérêt d'un Onguent Chinois (MEBO) dans le Maintient Local de l'Humidité. Bishara Journal des Plaies et Cicatrisation 2005;9:7–11.

Burn Pathophysiology

Theresa J. Nowak, CPT, RN, BSN, CCRN

KEYWORDS

• Burns • Burn pathophysiology • Inflammation • Burn injury
• Zones of injury

Burns affect more than 1.1 million people each year. Although this number has declined by over half since the 1960s, burns account for over 700,000 emergency department visits and 45,000 annual hospital admissions. Definitive treatment for burn victims is provided at 125 specialized burn centers in the nation.[1] According to the American Burn Association's National Burn Repository of 2010 (a compilation of data for the period 2000–2009), males made up 70% of burn admissions, and the average age of all admissions was 32 years. Seventy-one percent of admissions incurred burns equal to or less than a total body surface area (TBSA) of 10%, and the most common cause was fire/flame and scald. Scald injuries were most common in children, and fire/flame was more prevalent in the older population. Sixty-six percent of burns occurred at home or outside the workplace. In general, the probability of death from burn injury increased according to burn size, age, the presence of inhalation injury, and preexisting comorbidities. Inhalation injury alone increased likelihood of death by 25 times in patients under 60 years old with a TBSA less than 20%. Length of stay was dependent on TBSA. Surviving patients spent 1 day in the hospital per 1% burned. For patients who did not survive with a TBSA below 40%, their hospital stay was less than 3 weeks.[2]

Although the majority of burn injuries are survivable because of many medical advances over the years, basic burn identification and knowledge of burn pathophysiology remain crucial. In order to properly treat burn wounds, a provider must have a solid knowledge base in identification of burn wounds and the pathophysiology of the stress response and burn shock. This article highlights the anatomy of the skin and the zones of burn injury and introduces the different classifications of burn wounds. Finally, the pathophysiology of the stress response and burn shock are addressed.

BURN CENTER ADMISSION CRITERIA

Burn treatment requires specialized care during the initial injury and following discharge from the inpatient facility. Physicians, physician assistants, nurses, physical

The author has nothing to disclose.
DOD disclaimer: "The opinions or assertions contained herein are the private views of the author and are not to be construed as official or as reflecting the views of the Department of the Army or the Department of Defense."
United States Army Institute of Surgical Research, San Antonio, TX, USA
E-mail address: Theresa.j.nowak@us.army.mil

therapists, respiratory therapists, and nutritionists are just a few of the highly trained and specialized professionals within a burn center. The American Burn Association outlines patient requirements for admission to a burn center. The following burns meet referral criteria:

1. Partial thickness burns greater than 10% TBSA.
2. Burns that involve the face, hands, feet, genitalia, perineum, or major joints.
3. Third-degree burns in any age group.
4. Electrical burns, including lightning injury.
5. Chemical burns.
6. Inhalation injury.
7. Burn injury in patients with preexisting medical disorders that could complicate management, prolong recovery, or affect mortality.
8. Any patient with burns and concomitant trauma (such as fractures) in which the burn injury poses the greatest risk of morbidity or mortality. In such cases, if the trauma poses the greater immediate risk, the patient may be initially stabilized in a trauma center before being transferred to a burn unit. Physician judgment will be necessary in such situations and should be in concert with the regional medical control plan and triage protocols.
9. Burned children in hospitals without qualified personnel or equipment for the care of children.
10. Burn injury in patients who will require special social, emotional, or rehabilitative intervention.[3]

THE INTEGUMENTARY SYSTEM

In order to understand the pathophysiology of burns, the structure and function of normal skin must be revisited. The skin is the body's largest organ and serves many functions. These functions include fluid and electrolyte balance, temperature regulation, storage of fat, vitamin production, and protection against injury infection. It is composed of two layers, the epidermis and dermis (**Fig. 1**). The top layer, the epidermis, is the thinnest layer, measuring 0.05 mm (eyelids) to 1.0 mm (soles of feet). Thickness of skin depends on the dermis and varies with age, gender, and body location. The epidermis is composed of programmed cells, keratinocytes, which die and regenerate every 2 to 4 weeks. Keratinocytes flatten and harden as they die. The epidermis also contains melanocytes, which provide protection against ultraviolet radiation through the production of melanin. Melanocytes regenerate more slowly than keratinocytes, which can lead to permanent pigment changes when the skin begins to heal from a burn. The epidermis is also home to nerves that arise from the dermis. These nerves mediate the body's responses of pain and itching following a burn.[4]

Below the epidermis is the vascular and nervous section of the skin known as the dermis. This layer is thicker, ranging between 1 mm and 4 mm, and contains sensory nerves, blood vessels, sebaceous glands, eccrine sweat glands, apocrine sweat glands, and hair follicles that give rise in the epidermis.[1] The vascular networks of capillaries provide nutrients throughout the epidermis and dermis. Unlike the epidermis, the dermis heals by scarring and fibrosis instead of regeneration.

Underneath the dermis is a layer of subcutaneous tissue that is composed of adipose tissue. The adipose tissue, commonly referred to as fat, provides a layer of protection and insulation for the body.

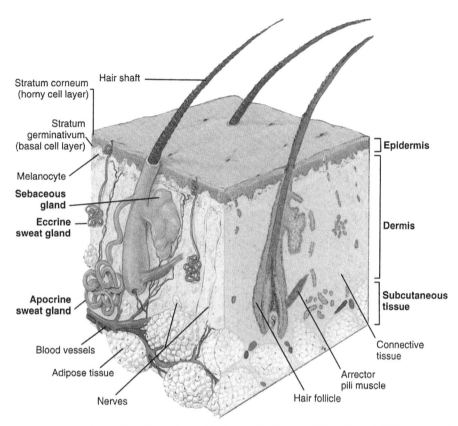

Stratum corneum
(horny cell layer)

Hair shaft

Stratum
germinativum
(basal cell layer)

Melanocyte

**Sebaceous
gland**

**Eccrine
sweat gland**

**Apocrine
sweat gland**

Blood vessels

Adipose tissue

Nerves

] Epidermis

Dermis

] **Subcutaneous
tissue**

Connective
tissue

Arrector
pili muscle

Hair follicle

Fig. 1. Layers of the skin. (*From* Stout LR. Burns. In: Carlson KK, editor. AACN: advanced critical care nursing. Canada: Saunders, Elsevier; 2009. p. 1215; with permission.)

ZONES OF BURN INJURY

There are multiple types of burns: thermal, chemical, electrical, radiation, friction, and freezing. Severity of burn depends on three factors: heat intensity, duration of exposure, and tissue conductance. Temperature and duration of contact have a synergistic effect. Cell necrosis occurs after 1 second of exposure to 156° F or 1 hour at 113° F.[4] Thermal burn injuries are the most common and are the main focus. The location of a thermal burn is divided into three zones (**Fig. 2**). The first zone is the most inner, the zone of coagulation. In this zone, blood circulation has ceased and there is vast cellular coagulation necrosis because this area obtained the most damage from extreme heat exposure. The cells are dead and will not regenerate independently. Therefore, this zone will require surgical excision and grafting.

The second zone of injury is the zone of stasis. This zone surrounds the zone of coagulation and is at high risk for cellular necrosis because circulation is greatly diminished. The viability of skin within this zone depends on proper fluid resuscitation and treatment for survival. Treatment within the first 24 to 72 hours is vital.[4] This zone of injury is the most challenging for a burn team to treat because it has the most potential to extend the zone of coagulation.

The third zone of injury is the zone of hyperemia. This zone borders the first two zones and is the least damaged because it was farthest from the source of injury. Skin

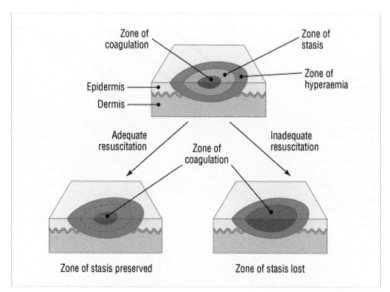

Fig. 2. Burn zones. (*From* Hettiaratchy S, Dziewulski P. ABC of burns; pathophysiology and types of burns. BMJ 2004;328:1427–9; with permission.)

within this zone responds to injury by releasing inflammatory mediators such as cytokines, causing vasodilation. Vasodilation allows nutrients to move to the area of injury to aid in recovery and removal of wastes. This zone is not structurally damaged and will regenerate.[5]

CLASSIFICATION OF BURN WOUNDS

Classification of burn wound depends on depth of injury and is diagnosed according to appearance of the skin. In this section, four main classifications of burn wounds and their appearance are discussed (**Fig. 3**).

The first classification is first-degree, also known as superficial. An example of this burn classification is sunburn. Like a sunburn, superficial burns are painful and red (no blisters present), because only the epidermis is affected. Recall from the previous section on skin that the epidermis is composed of regenerating cells, keratinocytes, and melanocytes. These cells are unique because they will spontaneously heal within 2 to 4 weeks. This burn will visibly heal within 3 to 6 days. These burns are painful because there are nerves present in this layer of skin.[4]

The second classification of burn wound is second-degree, with two subcategories, superficial partial-thickness and deep partial-thickness. Second-degree wounds affect the epidermis and extend into the dermis. Common causes of this burn type include limited exposure to hot liquid, flame, flash, or a chemical agent. Superficial partial-thickness burns extend through the epidermis and into the dermis. Such burns are painful, usually blister, and are red in color. These burns will usually heal within 10 to 14 days without scarring or surgery. On the other hand, deep partial-thickness burns extend through the epidermis and further into the dermis. These burns will likely require skin grafting because there is a distinct zone of coagulation. These burns are less moist, mottled, and pale and may or may not have blanching. Patients with this injury typically feel sensitivity to pressure because of the depth of the burns and subsequent damage to nerve endings.[1]

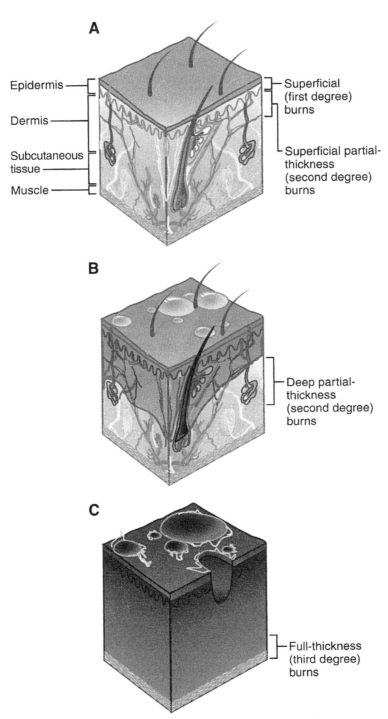

Fig. 3. Layers of the skin and depth of burn wound. (*A*) Superficial (first-degree) burn. (*B*) Deep partial-thickness (second-degree) burn. (*C*) Full-thickness (third-degree) burn. (*From* Stout LR. Burns. In: Carlson KK, editor. AACN: advanced critical care nursing. Canada: Saunders, Elsevier; 2009. p. 1224; with permission.)

The third classification of burns is third-degree, also known as full-thickness. Full thickness involves the entire epidermis and dermis and may extend into the subcutaneous fat. These burns will require surgical skin excision and grafting unless a very small percentage of skin is affected. The necrotic tissue is referred to as eschar and varies in thickness depending on length of exposure to the source. Full-thickness burns are nonblanching, dry, leathery, and pale. Vessels are thrombosed throughout, and only deep pressure can be felt. Healing time always depends on a variety of factors when the skin is excised and grafted. Healing grafts require ample nutrition, daily meticulous cleansing and debridement, and application of burn dressings within clean and sterile parameters to prevent infection.

The final burn classification known as fourth-degree is not routinely used in the United States. Fourth-degree classifies wounds that extend through the epidermis, dermis, and subcutaneous fat and down to bone, fascia, and tendons. Treatment of this burn often requires amputation (if it involves a limb), because the depth of the burn causes necrosis of all viable tissue, limiting grafting capabilities. Burns of this magnitude appear as charred.[1]

THE BODY'S STRESS RESPONSE

When a person is burned, the body immediately responds in a state of stress. This response is most commonly known as the "fight or flight" response. This response is a critical series of hormonal and physiologic responses that help a person deal with a stressful or life-threatening situation. It allows either flight to safety or fighting off the stressor.

Exposure to a stressful situation heightens emotions, causing the person to feel fear, terror, caution, and so on, ultimately activating the stress response. These emotions are interpreted in the brain's amygdala. Following interpretation, the amygdala automatically alerts the hypothalamus. The hypothalamus is the command center of the brain. It sends messages throughout the body via the autonomic nervous system (ANS). The ANS controls the body's involuntary functions such as breathing, heart rate, blood pressure, and dilation or constriction of blood vessels and small airways of the lungs. The ANS is subdivided into the sympathetic and parasympathetic nervous system. The sympathetic nervous system supplies the body with energy during the stress response (fight or flight), and the parasympathetic system slows the body down, also known as "rest or digest," when the danger has passed.[1]

After the amygdala sends a distress signal to the hypothalamus, the hypothalamus immediately responds in a state of alarm and activates the ANS. The ANS alerts the sympathetic nervous systemic via the adrenal glands. The adrenal glands secrete the hormones epinephrine and norepinephrine into the bloodstream. Epinephrine and norepinephrine circulate throughout the body, affecting it immensely. Epinephrine stimulates the heart to pump faster, causing an increase in blood pressure and heart rate. Blood flow increases to major organs and muscles. During this time respiratory rate is increased, and the lungs adapt to allow for more air to flow by dilating small airways. The increased respiratory rate enhances oxygen delivery to the brain, improving the person's attentiveness. In turn, the body's auditory and visual senses sharpen. Epinephrine also stimulates the release of glucose and fat from storage sites in the body to help maintain a constant level of energy. Norepinephrine increases metabolic activity and stimulates peripheral vasoconstriction, causing a decrease in urine output, slowing the digestive tract, and limiting blood flow to skin.[6]

Following the body's initial fight or flight response, the hypothalamus activates the hypothalamic-pituitary-adrenal (HPA) axis, the second element of the stress response. The HPA axis is composed of the hypothalamus, the pituitary gland, and the adrenal glands. The HPA axis allows the body to remain at a heightened level of alertness for an extended amount of time through the release of cortisol. The hypothalamus releases corticotrophin-releasing hormone to trigger the pituitary gland to release adrenocorticotropic hormone (ACTH). ACTH travels to the adrenal glands and subsequently releases cortisol. Cortisol increases blood glucose to help maintain the body's energy needs. When the stressful situation passes, the cortisol levels drop, stimulating the parasympathetic nervous system. The parasympathetic nervous system triggers the rest and digest period, signaling the end of the stress response. The adrenal glands also increase the amount of aldosterone circulating through the body. Aldosterone signals the kidneys to retain sodium, which further signals the body to retain water. In response, there is a loss of potassium, which functions as a negative feedback loop telling the body to decrease the release of aldosterone.[6]

TYING IT ALL TOGETHER

A burn injury instigates a myriad of internal changes. As mentioned previously, the body's initial instinct with a burn is the fight or flight response triggered by the ANS. After the initial burn insult has occurred and the rest and digest period has begun, the body enters into a state of burn shock.

Burn shock is unique because it presents as a combination of both distributive and hypovolemic shock.[6] Once a significant burn has occurred, the body releases inflammatory mediators, which are the bodily defense mechanisms to injury. These inflammatory mediators are released both systemically and locally to the damaged area. The most predominant mediators are bradykinin, histamine, prostaglandins, leukotrienes, and catecholamines.[7] Whereas mediators provide the body with defense against injury, they also can trigger a list of systemic responses that are harmful. The most harmful is hypovolemia.

The release of inflammatory mediators, primarily histamine, hinder capillary wall integrity, resulting in capillary leakage. This leakage pulls proteins and larger molecules from the intravascular space, decreasing the osmotic and hydrostatic pressure ultimately allowing fluid to escape. Alongside proteins, electrolytes and fluid from the intravascular space flow into the interstitium. These systemic changes result in the loss of circulating plasma volume, hemoconcentration, massive edema formation, decreased urine output, and depressed cardiovascular function. Edema formation usually peaks within 24 hours of burn injury.[7]

Besides histamine, bradykinin, prostaglandins, leukotrienes, and catecholamines have systemic and local effects that contribute to massive tissue edema formation and hypovolemia. Prostaglandins and leukotrienes contribute to the inflammatory response systemically by increasing microvascular permeability instigating edema formation. Bradykinins have a primarily local inflammatory effect. Also referred to as kinins, this mediator increases venule permeability. Last, catecholamines are released in large amounts following burn injury. Epinephrine and norepinephrine cause vasoconstriction of arterial microvessels, reducing capillary pressure. Reducing capillary pressure can limit edema formation and aid in interstitial fluid reabsorption by nonburned skin.[8]

Aside from massive edema formation, burn injury affects the cardiovascular, pulmonary, digestive, and renal systems most noticeably (**Fig. 4**). Following a massive burn, the most noticeable result is the body's hypermetabolic state. This is a direct result of increased oxygen consumption and metabolic rate instigated by heat loss. With hypovolemia there is less blood circulating throughout the body, resulting in

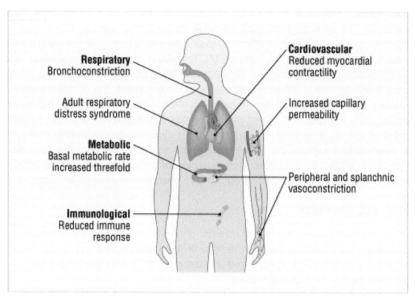

Fig. 4. Effects of burn injury on systems. (*From* Hettiaratchy S, Dziewulski P. ABC of burns; pathophysiology and types of burns. BMJ 2004;328:1427–9; with permission.)

decreased cardiac output and reduced venous return to the heart. In turn, edema formation worsens, and myocardial depression ensues because of a reduction in circulating oxygen.

The lungs, whether or not the patient sustained an inhalation injury, are susceptible to injury and illness. Any noninhalation burn patient may need intubation to protect the airway from edema, but all inhalation-positive burn patients will need intubation. Burn injuries can lead to acute lung injury and acute respiratory distress syndrome (ARDS). Both diseases originate from hypoxemia and other inflammatory factors that cause decreased lung compliance and result in bilateral lung infiltrates. ARDS is the most prominent insult to the lungs. Associated causes of ARDS are the presence of smoke inhalation, pneumonia, or mediators of sepsis and inflammation.[8]

Major pathophysiologic changes in the gastrointestinal tract that affect normal function include decreased absorption, decreased mobility, mucosal atrophy, and increased intestinal permeability. These abnormalities are caused by hypoperfusion of the gut. The result of these physiologic abnormalities is translocation of bacteria, stomach and duodenal stress ulceration, and decreased pH levels. The patient is at high risk for infection when these issues ensue. Therefore, a key to prevention of gut dysfunction is early administration of enteral nutrition and mediation of gut acidic levels by administration of antacid medication.[9]

During initial burn treatment and throughout hospitalization, caregivers rely on renal function to monitor fluid resuscitation and overall fluid status of the patient. However, the effects of burn shock are devastating on the kidneys. Decreased blood flow and vasoconstriction limit the kidney's functionality, increasing the risk for acute renal failure. Once renal blood flow has decreased and acute renal failure occurs, damage sustained by the kidneys is often irreversible. Mortality is 50% for those diagnosed with acute renal failure.[9]

REFERENCES

1. Stout LR. Burns. In: Carlson KK, editor. AACN: advanced critical care nursing. Canada: Saunders, Elsevier; 2009. p. 1212–60.
2. American Burn Association. Summary of findings. National Burn Repository 2010. Available at: http://www.ameriburn.org/. Accessed April 21, 2011.
3. American Burn Association. Burn center referral criteria. Available at: http://www.ameriburn.org/. Accessed May 10, 2011.
4. Heimbach DM, Gibran NS, Pham TN. Evaluation of the burn wound: management decisions. In: Herndon DN, editor. Total burn care. 3rd edition. China: Saunders, Elsevier; 2007. p. 119–26.
5. Evers LH, Bhavsar D, Mailander P. The biology of burn injury: review article. Exp Dermatol 2010;19:777–83.
6. Siedlecki SL. Pain and sedation. In: Carlson KK, editor. AACN: advanced critical care nursing. Canada: Saunders, Elsevier; 2009. p. 44–87.
7. Latenser BA. Critical care of the burn patient: the first 48 hours: concise definitive review. Crit Care Med 2009;37(10):2819–26.
8. Kramer GC, Lund T, Beckum OK. Pathophysiology of burn shock and burn edema. In: Herndon DN, editor. Total burn care. 3rd edition. China: Saunders, Elsevier; 2007. p. 93–102.
9. Wolf SE. Critical care in the severely burned: organ support and management of complications. In: Herndon DN, editor. Total burn care. 3rd edition. China: Saunders, Elsevier; 2007. p. 454–76.

Caring for the Burn Patient: The Perioperative Nurse

Bonnie A. Jackson, RN, MSN, CCNS-C[a],*, Mary Sueltenfuss, RN, BSN, NLC[b]

KEYWORDS

- Perioperative nursing • Burn care

Imagine traveling through an extended hallway accompanied by strangers dressed in green garments speaking a language you have never heard before. Now imagine traveling that same path, but this time with a confident nurse alongside you translating the language for you and advocating for you during the journey. For the burn patient, especially one who has suffered severe burns, the hospital environment can be a daunting experience. Burn patients often feel afraid and intensely vulnerable. The perioperative nurse has the unique opportunity to empower and positively impact patients and their outcome by assisting and guiding them through this challenging and difficult process. The skilled perioperative nurse has available a wide variety of talents and tools such as critical thinking, problem-solving, technical expertise, and genuine, compassionate caring.

The role of the perioperative nurse encompasses three phases of the patient's surgical or procedural journey: the preoperative, intraoperative, and postoperative periods. Each phase of the experience has its own unique aspects and priorities, but all are designed to be carefully interwoven and in concert with each other while moving the patient through the process toward a desired outcome or goal.

During the preoperative phase the nursing tasks focus on providing preoperative education and teaching, monitoring of the patient's physical and emotional well-being, and assisting the surgeon and anesthesia provider with the informed consent process. This preoperative phase is where the patient is readied for surgery including being given a thorough preoperative assessment that may include history and physical examination, laboratory studies, radiographs, and review of any medications, blood transfusions, or equipment ordered.

The opinions or assertions contained herein are the private views of the author and are not to be construed as official or as reflecting the views of the Department of the Army or the Department of Defense.

a United States Army Institute of Surgical Research-Battlefield Medicine, 3698 Chambers Pass, Fort Sam Houston, TX 78234-6315, USA
b Department of Anesthesiology, United States Army Institute of Surgical Research and Army Burn Center, Brooke Army Medical Center, 3400 Rawley East Chambers Avenue, Fort Sam Houston, TX 78234, USA
* Corresponding author.
E-mail address: bonnie.ann.jackson@us.army.mil

The roles and responsibilities of the perioperative nurse evolve as the patient is transported from the inpatient room or the outpatient preparation area to the holding area and ultimately into the operating room. The nurse continues to stand ready as an advocate for the patient, even when that patient is unconscious and under the effects of anesthesia. Roles that an intraoperative nurse can assume in the operating room include functioning as a circulating nurse, scrub nurse in the sterile field, or first assistant to the surgeon.

Once the surgery has been completed, the patient is moved to the postanesthesia care unit (PACU) to recover under the vigilant watch of the PACU nurse. Assessing the sixth vital sign, for pain, and administering the appropriate medications are integral to the PACU nurse's skill set. The airway and respirations are intently monitored to assure a patent airway and adequate oxygenation. Fluids are titrated and administered while the patient is continually monitored for hemodynamic stability. All physiologic functions are monitored for postoperative response. The PACU nurse performs frequent neurologic assessments (neuro checks), evaluating levels of consciousness, sensation, and readiness for discharge from the PACU.

The common thread woven through all three phases of perioperative nursing is the caring and compassion that the nurse provides. From the very first interaction with the patient and/or family the nurse skillfully begins to construct the foundation of a trusting relationship. The perioperative nurse applies Watson's caring theory,[1] which dates back to the 1970s and is used today. Watson believed nurses share their spiritual energy and humanistic approach, based on morals and values, with their patients in each interaction. Nursing demonstrates respect and compassion for the patient through nurses' unique circumstances. Watson believed that the patient perceives the love and caring the nurse dispenses. With this growing and dynamic aspect introduced into the patient-nurse relationship, the patient is more amenable to asking questions and more secure in voicing fears and concerns. When the perioperative nurse demonstrates unconditional acceptance, difficult conversations can be honestly and respectfully explored, such as the do not resuscitate order and the completion of a living will or an advanced directive. Patients become engaged and communication becomes more effective as the nurse empowers them.

The trusting and caring interaction of the perioperative nurse holistically embraces the patient and can fortify the burn patient's commitment to self-healing and self-growth. Burn patients face a multitude of challenges, beginning with the initial injury and insult, to the rigors of ongoing pain and, for many, an altered self-image. Ultimately, the positive interaction may translate into improved patient outcomes as well as improved patient and provider satisfaction.

One of the most powerful tools perioperative nurses possess is the one they innately carry within themselves. Like breathing in and breathing out, genuine caring and respect and unconditional acceptance can provide a healing balm that enables a burn patient to muster inner resources. Florence Nightingale was quoted as saying, "It is the surgeon who saves a person's life. . .it is the nurse who helps this person live."[1]

We have gone to school, become proficient in our technical skills, and learned to speak the language. Now we enter the hospital room and are automatically perceived to be the confident guide that comes beside our burn patients to help them navigate their new, unfamiliar, and intimidating journey. As we reach into our tool kit and pull out our needle, we must thread it with the twine of caring compassion. It is our duty to skillfully weave caring compassion into the fabric of our patient-nurse relationship. Perioperative nurses see the individual, not just the scar. We see the person, not just the burn. When questioned about why we do what we do, the simple but profound reply is, "Because we care." We spell nursing C-A–R–I–N–G.

REFERENCE

1. Watson J. Human caring science. A theory of nursing. 2nd edition. Sudbury (MA): Jones & Bartlett; 2011. A new revised edition of Human Science and Human Care. Originally published in 1985.

Perioperative Anesthetic Considerations for Burn Patients

Christopher V. Maani, MD, MC, US Army[a],*, Jacob J. Hansen, DO[b],
Patricia A. Fortner, RN, MSN, MEd, CNOR[c], Leopoldo C. Cancio, MD[b],
Peter A. DeSocio, DO[d]

KEYWORDS

• Perioperative • Burn patients • Anesthesia • Nursing

One of the challenges faced by military healthcare providers in Operation Iraqi Freedom (OIF) and Operation Enduring Freedom (OEF) is the treatment of severely burned Wounded Warriors and local civilians. As with the management of other combat-related injuries sustained during the overseas contingency operations, modern-day burn care reaps the benefits of recent advancements in evacuation times from point of injury through Landstuhl Regional Medical Center in Germany to the US Army Institute of Surgical Research (USAISR) Burn Center at Brooke Army Medical Center, Fort Sam Houston, Texas. The USAISR Burn Center is the Department of Defense's only military facility treating severely burned soldiers. The burn center has a dedicated operating suite (operating room [OR]) and OR staff to include an independent anesthesia department and a surgical team consisting of 11 surgeons and six physician assistants. The burn center also provides care to patients of the US Department of Veterans Affairs, several federal agencies, and civilians in the south Texas region.

Burn patients have perioperative anesthesia concerns that are distinct from other surgical populations. These issues require consideration and planning by the surgical team and the anesthesia provider (anesthesiologist or nurse anesthetist) in order to

The opinions or assertions contained in this article are the private views of the authors, and are not to be construed as reflecting the views of the United States Army or the Department of Defense.

[a] Department of Anesthesiology, United State Army Institute of Surgical Research and Army Burn Center, Brooke Army Medical Center, 3400 Rawley East Chambers Avenue, Fort Sam Houston, TX 78234, USA

[b] Medical Corps, United States Army Burn Center, United States Army Institute of Surgical Research, 3698 Chambers Pass, Fort Sam Houston, TX 78234-6315, USA

[c] United States Army Nurse Corps CR Darnall Army Medical Center, Fort Hood, TX 76544, USA

[d] Department of Anesthesia, The Ohio State University Medical Center, N411 Doan Hall, 410 West 10th Avenue, Columbus, OH 43210, USA

* Corresponding author.

E-mail address: Christopher.Maani@us.army.mil

obtain optimal outcomes. The USAISR Clinical Division consists of 16 intensive care unit (ICU) beds and 24 intermediate-care patient beds. During a 3-year period (Jan 2008–Dec 2010), the Army Burn Center has treated more than 168 severely burned soldiers from OIF in Iraq and OEF in Afghanistan, with total admissions of 1145 patients (Bonnie Jackson, RN, personal communication, 2010). Of these admissions, 177 patients (15.4%) had an average total body surface area (TBSA) burn greater than 20%, compared with 5.3% from the National Burn Repository.[1] The experience gained by the authors at the USAISR Burn Center guides the discussion on these pages, but the intent is to shepherd the provision of burn care in medical settings outside of established burn centers such as the Combat Support Hospital and other austere or deployed settings. This article is written to accompany and chaperone OR personnel with limited experience caring for burn patients and discusses anesthetic and perioperative considerations that may be encountered in these patients.

ACUTE INJURY

The first 24- to 48-hour period after a major burn is commonly referred to as the resuscitation phase. During this time the patient will be resuscitated with intravenous (IV) fluids in an attempt to optimize intravascular volume and urine output. This procedure usually results in IV fluid volumes much larger than typical maintenance rates. There are several formulas used to guide hourly infusion rates, but the therapeutic goal is usually determined by titrating to maintain urine output between 0.5 and 1cc/kg/h.[2,3] Overresuscitation should be avoided because it will lead to increased edema and related complications.[4] During this phase the patient may require escharotomy (an incision into a burn eschar in order to lessen tension on the underlying tissue [**Fig. 1**]) or fasciotomy (an incision into the fascia in order to relieve compartmental pressure within the fascia) to preserve perfusion to extremities or to allow ventilation. Less commonly a decompressive laparotomy is required to treat intraabdominal hypertension. Blood transfusion is not typically required during the resuscitative phase because there is limited blood loss and the patient's hematocrit is normal to high, assuming he or she has not lost blood from other traumatic injuries and may be hemoconcentrated. Nonburn injuries may also dictate other operative procedures during this phase. Examples include acute neurosurgical management of head injuries and surgical stabilization of severe orthopedic trauma. In general, when performing procedures during the resuscitation phase, it is helpful to keep in mind the goal of maintaining organ perfusion as demonstrated by a minimally acceptable urine output rather than volume loading to intravascular euvolemia.

Respiratory failure is commonly encountered during the resuscitation phase, and anesthesia providers may be called on during this period to intubate the patient. As burn size increases, the risk of generalized edema, to include airway edema, increases as well. This increase places the burn patient at increased risk of airway obstruction for TBSA burns of 40% or greater, even in the absence of inhalation injury. Additionally, the patient with damage to the respiratory tract may require intubation regardless of the size of the burn. Generally, intubation should be done earlier rather than later in such a patient, but it is usually an urgent rather than emergent procedure, and time should be taken to optimize the preparation for the procedure and safety of the patient. The decision of whether or not to intubate a given patient in the acute setting often requires considerable judgment. Subtle clues such as a subjective change in the patient's voice may tip the decision. The conduct of acute phase intubations generally does not require any unusual considerations beyond those of any other trauma patient. If the decision is delayed until the patient is in respiratory distress, there is a high risk of significant hemodynamic compromise during intubation. A large endotracheal tube (at least 7.5

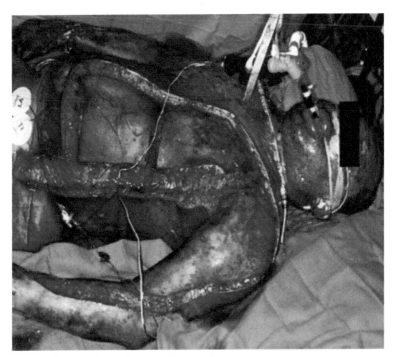

Fig. 1. Burn escharotomies and severe airway edema.

for women, 8.0 for men) is preferred to accommodate respiratory care and the likely need for bronchoscopy. However, airway edema may compromise the ability to place a larger endotracheal tube. In such a circumstance, the smaller tube may be exchanged under controlled circumstances, even in the OR if necessary.

GENERAL BURN CARE

A more in-depth discussion detailing general burn care is presented elsewhere in this issue; however, some pertinent attributes affecting perioperative care are considered here. Nonsurgical care of burn wounds is continuously evolving. Topical antibiotic creams and solutions are used on some partial- or full-thickness burns. Silver sulfadiazine (Silvadene) and mafenide acetate (Sulfamylon) are the most commonly used agents. Silvadene is considered less painful to apply but does not penetrate intact burn eschar. Silvadene may also cause leukopenia, typically in the first few days of use.[5] Sulfamylon penetrates burn eschar but can be painful to apply. Sulfamylon is a carbonic anhydrase inhibitor, which may be associated with metabolic acidosis.[6,7] In patients with large burns or renal failure who are treated exclusively with Sulfamylon, a hyperchloremic metabolic acidosis is occasionally seen that may be attributable to Sulfamylon and may not resolve until the drug is withdrawn. Silver nitrate is also effective but not frequently used because its use is somewhat labor intensive and it lacks superiority over other agents.

EXCISION AND GRAFTING

Full-thickness burns, unless very small, must be treated with excision and grafting. Partial-thickness burns may require excision and grafting or may be treated nonsurgically, depending on depth, size, and location. Excision of burned skin and placing skin grafts is the bulk of burn surgery. There is some controversy over the exact timing of this surgery, but most centers will conduct the first operation within a few days of the patient being burned. Over the years the definition of early excision has changed somewhat, with early becoming progressively earlier. Originally, burns were treated nonoperatively until full-thickness eschar had been removed and granulation tissue had formed, a process that could take weeks. Currently, an excision within 48 hours of injury would be considered early. Some surgeons will operate as soon as possible, whereas others prefer to wait 48 hours to allow the patient to complete initial resuscitation.[8,9] There is no clearly optimal timing for all patients.[9,10] Likewise, some surgeons will restrict the scope of the operation to 20% TBSA. Other burn surgeons prefer to remove as much of the burn as possible during the first surgery, but excisions of more than 10% to 20% by inexperienced surgeons place the patient at risk of excessive blood loss and are discouraged.

Excision may be either tangential, in which the burn is excised in thin layers using a hand dermatome (eg, Humby, Blair, Brown, Braithwaite, Goulian) until unburned tissue is reached, or fascial, in which all skin and underlying fat is removed down to fascia, usually by using an electrocautery device. Tangential excision generally produces a better functional and cosmetic result. Fascial excision is preferred for contaminated burns and for those that extend into the fat. Whichever method is chosen, these procedures can be quite bloody, with blood loss varying from 123 to 387 cc for each 1% TBSA excised.[11–13] Intraoperative blood loss varies with several factors. Less blood loss may be associated with fascial excisions, fresh burns, and more centrally located burns. Greater degrees of blood loss are typically seen with older burns, infected burns, and extremity burns.[13] The use of tourniquets or various topical hemostatic agents may reduce blood loss substantially.[12]

Harvesting of the skin graft may produce considerable blood loss itself, especially if the scalp is harvested. Infiltration of epinephrine solution (eg, via a Pitkin device) in the area to be harvested can reduce or eliminate this blood loss.[14] Alternatively, subdermal clysis can be performed by injection of saline or lactated Ringer's solution with 1 to 2 mg of epinephrine per liter using, for example, a 60-mL syringe and an 18-gauge needle or spinal needle. Other combinations of vasoconstrictors in crystalloid solutions may be equally effective. Postoperatively, most patients report that the site of graft harvest is much more painful than the site of the excised burn. For this reason regional anesthesia may be part of the anesthetic plan.

OR SETUP

For OR setup, all standard equipment should be present and machine checks done as for a routine case. The room should be heated to 90°F or as close to that as possible. Commonly the patient's entire body must be exposed, limiting the usefulness of warming blankets. Burn-injured patients often present with difficult airway challenges. Some alternative means of securing the airway beyond direct laryngoscopy should be immediately available. A rapid infusion system capable of warming and infusing blood at 100 to 200 mL/min should be available. Blood products should be immediately available, although the amount is highly variable by specific circumstances. For large excisions, 10 to 20 units of packed red cells may be needed over several hours. Platelets and plasma are often required for larger excisions even if the patient starts with normal coagulation. Additional IV and/or central line supplies should be in the room.

PREOPERATIVE EVALUATION

Some burn patients will be extremely ill when scheduled for surgery. The anesthesia provider may discuss with the surgeon and ICU team the risks and benefits of proceeding to the OR when planning for these patients; however, the concept of the patient being "too sick" to go to the OR does not apply to the casualty who may not improve until the burn is removed. In cases of abdominal compartment syndrome or chest eschar inhibiting ventilation, surgery can make the patient much better immediately. The question to ask is whether there is a problem that can clearly be improved with nonsurgical treatment. If the answer is no, then the patient should not be delayed from going to the OR for needed surgery.

In addition to the standard preoperative evaluation, following are several areas that deserve extra attention in burn patients.

Airway

Patients with topical antimicrobials on their face may present difficulty with mask ventilation. A standard hand towel may be used to give the hands additional traction on the face, and the possibility of using a two-handed mask technique should be considered. Dressings may need to be removed to achieve an adequate mask seal. Patients in the acute portion of their care may have a tracheostomy. When the patient is no longer ventilator-dependent, the surgeons may wish to remove the tracheostomy tube in a patient who may require more surgical procedures. This decision requires individualized consideration of the risks and benefits to a particular patient and should be discussed in a team approach. Patients who are further out from their injury may develop scarring that limits mouth opening or neck extension. These features should be evident from routine examination and may indicate a plan that does not rely on a laryngoscope. For patients who will be intubated in the OR, securing the endotracheal tube often requires an alternative to adhesive tape. Cloth ties are commonly used, and suturing to a tooth is another viable option. Nasal intubation with cloth ties around the nasal septum is also quite effective.

Pulmonary

The oxygen concentration (FIO_2), ventilator pressures, and arterial blood gases (ABG) are useful in evaluating pulmonary issues. Burn patients routinely have higher-than-normal minute ventilation.[6] High FIO_2 and ventilator pressures combined with a poor ABG indicate possible difficulty in the OR. Patients with inhalation injuries frequently produce plugs or clots that can obstruct an endotracheal tube. This problem is especially concerning in a patient who is placed in a prone position. The combination of marginal lung performance, clot production, and prone position can result in a rapidly fatal loss of airway and/or hemodynamic collapse. The anesthesia team should have a plan for dealing with an obstructed tube beforehand, regardless of patient position, and communicate that plan to the rest of the OR crew. Very ill patients may need to remain on an ICU ventilator rather than the anesthesia ventilator or workstation, and this needs to be discussed with the respiratory therapy and surgical teams. In this case the anesthetic plan may require a total IV anesthetic (TIVA). Patients with high ventilator pressures and high inspired oxygen levels may desaturate rapidly when disconnected from their ventilator even briefly. This possibility should be considered when planning transportation of the patient.

Circulation

Patients who survive a major burn and the subsequent burn shock period have essentially passed a stress test. These patients should not require further cardiac evaluation except in unusual circumstances. A large burn frequently results in a rise in troponin, even in patients who do not have cardiac disease.[15] Burn patients are typically hyperdynamic and may remain so for weeks or months after their injury. Heart rates in adults of 110 to 120 are typical.[16] If a patient is hypotensive early in resuscitation, intravascular volume is frequently inadequate; later in the course afterload is more commonly the cause of hypotension, but either or both may be present. The patient will frequently require blood transfusion during excision. Knowing the hematocrit at the start of the procedure will help guide the timing and volume of blood products. Very sick patients with multiorgan dysfunction may require platelets or plasma, as will patients undergoing large excisions. Most patients are treated with some form of thromboprophylaxis. This will be a consideration if nerve blocks are planned.

Neurologic

The primary neurologic issues are pain control and sedation. Patients may be receiving large doses of narcotic or sedative drugs and yet remain surprisingly awake.[16] Verifying the patient's level of consciousness and drug doses in the previous 12 hours can help guide the amounts to be needed in the OR.

Vascular Access

An intact 18-gauge IV is sufficient in most cases, although patients with significant burn injury usually have a central line. If a multilumen central line is not available, a second large-bore IV is helpful if blood products or high volumes of fluids are anticipated. An cordis or introducer may be needed during the most extensive excisions. Some planning is required with smaller lines. Fluid or blood may need to be started earlier if multiple large-bore access sites are not available. An arterial line can be useful for larger excisions, to permit both monitoring and frequent laboratory assays. An arterial line may be indicated if the surgical plan leaves no suitable site for a noninvasive blood pressure cuff, or if the surgery is likely to result in significant hemodynamic instability. Placement of all lines must be made with the surgical plan in mind. Placing a line in or near an area to be excised or harvested should only be done when there are no better alternatives. Catheters are prepped into the surgical field when necessary. Even peripheral IV catheters are routinely secured with sutures or staples, because burn creams or surgical preparation solutions can render tape useless.

Nutrition

Nutrition is very important in healing and must be considered when holding enteral nutrition prior to surgery. A gastric tube may be used for aspiration of stomach contents immediately prior to taking a patient to the OR. For patients with feeding tubes beyond the pylorus, feeding may be continued until transport to the OR. There is some controversy about the need to stop feeding even then. The reason for stopping feeds in the OR is that the patients frequently are treated with vasopressors during and after surgery, which places them at risk of intestinal ischemia. Patients who are eating should generally be allowed to do so until 6 hours prior to their surgical time.

Drips and Drugs

Patients may require multiple infusions, especially in the ICU. Generally any infusion that is not absolutely necessary is stopped prior to transport to the OR. This minimizes the equipment required during transport and reduces the chance of errors, eg in regard to concentrated electrolyte solutions.

Preoperative antibiotics are frequently delayed or overlooked. It is important to verify that any antibiotics ordered have been given and that all on the operative team are aware.

IN THE OR

Once the patient has been transported to the OR, the next step is induction of anesthesia. Consideration should be given to induction on the patient's bed if movement is especially painful or if the patient will be positioned prone. Standard monitor placement and induction are generally straightforward, with a few exceptions. Monitor placement may be limited by injuries and dressings. Standard electrocardiograph lead placement is rarely essential, and leads may be placed where space can be found. Ordinary leads may not stick to burn patients but may be stapled in place after induction. The practice of using noninvasive blood pressure cuffs over burned and dressed extremities or full-thickness burns is discouraged. Arterial lines are sometimes needed for hemodynamic monitoring when limited body surface area is available.[17] Creativity may be needed in placing a pulse oximeter. Other than fingers and toes, the ears, nose, lips, forehead, and hard palate are some of the sites that may be successful. Exhaled carbon dioxide (CO_2) monitoring is essential in burn patients and is a reliable indicator of adequate ventilation as well as a rough guide to cardiac output, and it is the monitor least likely to fail in these patients. Temperature monitoring is almost always used. Inability to maintain a temperature of 36°C warrants maximal effort to warm the patient. A Foley catheter should be used in most cases. Movement of patients to or from the operating table is a high-risk period for the inadvertent removal of lines or tubes. Several people may be involved in this movement, and one of them should be identified to ensure lines and tubes are in position for movement.

Induction of anesthesia usually involves muscle relaxant drugs. Succinylcholine is widely recognized as being contraindicated in burn patients. Succinylcholine is safe for the first 24 hours after a burn, but beyond that period and for up to a year after healing it may cause a dramatic and fatal hyperkalemia.[18] Nondepolarizing muscle relaxants such as rocuronium or vecuronium are regularly used in burn patients with the understanding that they will require larger doses and will not last as long.[19] The exception to that rule is mivacurium, which lasts as long as or longer in burned patients than in nonburned patients.[20] Some patients develop a hyperreflexia that is commonly elicited when lifting a leg. This reaction can produce jerking that only stops with muscle relaxation. Aside from that possibility, muscle relaxants are generally not required beyond intubation.

Burn patients may be resistant to opiates, especially if they have been given large doses for several days, but they generally respond normally to the usual induction agents. The other drug response that is altered in burn patients is the response to catecholamines. They may require doses of phenylephrine (or other vasopressors) considerably higher than unburned patients to achieve similar results. Likewise, patients in burn shock (ie, large TBSA burns, first 24 hours) are at greater risk for significant, profound, and protracted hypotension upon induction with any agent capable of myocardial depression.

Patients who do not require an ICU ventilator may be given inhalational anesthesia. Potent inhalation agents supplemented with opiates work well for most patients. If a TIVA technique is chosen, propofol and ketamine supplemented by opiates work well. For patients with a large blood loss the propofol infusion may need to be decreased to very low rates even in well-resuscitated patients.[21] Ketamine has been a traditional choice in burn patients and works well either as a supplement to other IV agents or as the main anesthetic agent itself.[22] Emergence delirium is seldom an issue in critically ill ICU patients who are generally maintained on sedatives for days after their surgery. Despite its reputation for bizarre dreams, long-term psychological effects have not been documented with ketamine.[23]

Blood loss during the excision portion may be dramatic with loss of 1 to 2 L not uncommonly in a short period of time. Large excisions may feature loss of 5 L or more over the course of a few hours. When to transfuse is a decision that must be based on individual circumstances. Young healthy adults can easily tolerate a hematocrit of 20 or even less. Once the hematocrit drops below 18, patients typically become hypotensive and poorly responsive to vasopressors. Acidosis renders catecholaminergic vasopressors less effective, so vasopressin may be preferred in such a circumstance.[24] Older, less fit patients may be less tolerant of anemia. As a general rule, if the patient is hypotensive it is rarely wrong to initiate red blood cell transfusion while investigating the cause, especially if he or she is not responding well to fluid and phenylephrine. The quality of IV access and speed of blood loss will also influence the timing of transfusion. Some patients will require multiple units of packed red blood cells in a short period of time. This procedure may lead to decreased ionized calcium in the patient's blood and need for IV replacement.[25,26] The need for non–red cell blood products varies considerably from case to case and is usually driven by laboratory values, clinically observed bleeding, and the judgment of the staff. Recombinant activated factor VIIa has been occasionally used in cases involving large blood loss, but at present there are no data to prove that it is helpful.[27,28]

For larger excisions or unstable patients, frequent blood gasses may be helpful. The base deficit and hematocrit will guide the choice and amount of fluids used. Venous blood gasses may be used for this purpose if an arterial line is not in place. Urine output or lack thereof may also guide volume replacement. It is not uncommon to require vasopressors to maintain adequate blood pressure after surgery has begun. This requirement may be due to the release of endotoxins or other factors during excision of the wound. Vasopressin, norepinephrine, epinephrine, and phenylephrine are commonly used with effectiveness that varies from patient to patient. Care must be taken to ensure that anemia or hypovolemia is not the cause of hypotension before relying on vasopressors to maintain blood pressure.

If blood loss gets ahead of the resuscitation during surgery, it may be necessary to ask the surgeon to stop while the anesthesiologist or anesthetist transfuses to catch up. The basic first aid rule of holding pressure to stop bleeding can be effective. Epinephrine-soaked laparotomy sponges may be used to assist in hemostasis. Patients tend not to show a significant systemic response to the epinephrine in such an application.[12] Patients may receive several milligrams of subcutaneous epinephrine from subdermal clysis solution also without change of heart rate or blood pressure. In major cases the patient may receive several liters of fluid by clysis, which will be mobilized over the following 24 hours along with crystalloids that have been given intravenously. This volume must be considered when making decisions such as whether to extubate a patient after surgery.

After skin grafts are placed they may be dressed with a negative pressure dressing or conventional gauze dressings. At this point protecting the graft from shearing is important. If the patient is to be extubated, a smooth, pain-free wake-up will help prevent patient thrashing that may shear the grafts. If intubation is maintained, adequate sedative should be assured as the anesthetic gas is eliminated. Narcotic should be titrated to respiratory rate. As noted earlier, patients may require large doses.

POSTOPERATIVE CARE

ICU patients are transported to the ICU postoperatively, where the surgeon or ICU team will resume care. Patients should be monitored during this transport, and frequently they require supplemental oxygen and/or ventilator assistance. Once in the ICU room, the anesthesia provider must ensure that the patient is efficiently transferred from transport monitors to the ICU monitors. If it was necessary to start any vasopressors during the procedure or if the patient has been unstable, the anesthesia provider should ensure through proper report and turnover that the physician and nurse responsible for the patient in the ICU are present and are aware of those issues.

Ward patients may be taken to the recovery room and treated in the standard fashion for postanesthesia care. Patients with negative pressure dressings in place should be reconnected to suction without delay. Pain control usually requires treatment with opiates. Choice of opioid or other analgesic medications should be guided on an individual basis. Meperidine is not used because of potential for accumulation of toxic metabolites.[29] Methadone has also been used successfully, sometimes when other opiates have failed.[30]

OUT-OF-OR PROCEDURES

Burn patients often require wound care that may be quite painful. Surgeons will commonly attempt to treat these patients with a combination of benzodiazepines and opiates. Some patients cannot tolerate their care without more profound acute pain control. Wound care procedures are often done in a shower room. Sometimes this procedure may involve removing large adherent dressings or debridement of wounds. By performing aggressive wound care, some patients may avoid having to come to the OR.

There are numerous acceptable regimens for pain control in this situation. Choosing a plan that is familiar and comfortable for the anesthesia provider is probably more important than any particular drug selection. Commonly used medications include propofol, dexmedetomidine, and ketamine.

Airway control remains a primary concern in this scenario. Patients frequently require jaw lift to maintain spontaneous ventilation, especially after a bolus dose, but apnea is rare if opiates have not been added. These procedures are routinely performed without need for positive pressure ventilation or supplemental oxygen. Pulse oximetry is sufficient monitoring for most patients in this situation. Exhaled CO_2 monitoring can also be reassuring if it is available. Additional monitors may be considered based on individual patient issues, and one must always be prepared to provide advanced airway interventions and resuscitation if necessary.

ELECTRIC INJURIES

Patients with electric injury commonly have a superimposed thermal injury if the electrical current has ignited their clothing. There may be extensive underlying tissue destruction beyond the obvious contact point, especially with high-voltage injury.[31] Patients with electric injuries may be monitored in a burn ICU for 24 hours to observe for cardiac arrhythmias; however, malignant cardiac arrhythmias are rare.[32,33] Muscle destruction is common with electric injury, and monitoring renal and electrolyte abnormalities is mandatory. This possibility must be considered when planning for and implementing intraoperative resuscitative strategies as well as monitoring to include point-care tests. For example, patients with gross myoglobinuria merit resuscitation targeted to a higher urine output goal of 70 to 100 mL/h.

NONTHERMAL SKIN DISEASES

Any injury or disease that causes a significant loss of skin may be suitable for treatment in a burn unit. One of the most common disorders is toxic epidermal necrolysis syndrome (TENS). TENS has a reported 30% to 50% mortality.[34–36] The disease causes a partial-thickness skin injury that may also involve the mucosal membranes. The disease does not usually require skin grafting, but the anesthesia provider may be involved for airway issues. An important consideration is that mucous membranes may slough and cause bleeding with manipulation. Direct laryngoscopy in a TENS patient may result in bleeding sufficient to obscure the view of the airway. The first attempt at laryngoscopy may provide the only good view, and fiberoptic bronchoscopy may be difficult or impossible afterwards. This possibility should be considered when planning to secure the airway. TENS patients may also produce plugs that can acutely obstruct an endotracheal tube.

Other skin disorders may be treated in a burn unit from time to time but rarely pose an issue not already considered in the care of burn patients.

SUMMARY

Burn patients often return to the OR multiple times over the course of ensuing weeks to years after their initial traumatic injury. They make up one of the most challenging populations cared for by perioperative providers and anesthesiology teams alike. These brave patients remain physically and mentally tough despite difficult airways, poor IV access, hypermetabolic states, nutritional challenges, hemodynamic instability, frequent surgeries, and painful rehabilitation. Provision of care to this select population requires knowledge of and preparation for many specific issues as discussed herein. This scenario provides an opportunity for clinical continuity that anesthesia providers and perioperative nursing care teams seldom have with other patient cohorts, as well as the satisfaction of seeing patients progress from being critically ill to recovered and functional. With proper planning and close coordination with the burn care team, these patients can be cared for effectively, compassionately, and safely.

ACKNOWLEDGMENTS

The authors would like to extend special appreciation to Bonnie Jackson (USAISR Burn Program manager) and Mary Sueltenfuss (USAISR Pain Task Area Clinical Research Coordinator) for their contributions to this article and for assistance in manuscript preparation.

REFERENCES

1. Latenser B. National Burn Repository 2006: a ten-year review. J Burn Care Res 2007;28(5):635–58.
2. Monafo WW. Initial management of burns. N Engl J Med 1996;335(21):1581–6.
3. Warden GD. Burn shock resuscitation. World J Surg 1992;16(1):16–23.

4. Ivy ME, Atweh NA, Palmer J, et al. Intra-abdominal hypertension and abdominal compartment syndrome in burn patients. J Trauma 2000;49(3):387–91.
5. Jarrett F, Ellerbe S, Demling R. Acute leukopenia during topical burn therapy with silver sulfadiazine. Am J Surg 1978;135(6):818–9.
6. Petroff PA, Hander EW, Mason AD Jr. Ventilatory patterns following burn injury and effect of sulfamylon. J Trauma 1975;15(8):650–6.
7. Asch MJ, White MG, Pruitt BA Jr. Acid base changes associated with topical Sulfamylon therapy: retrospective study of 100 burn patients. Ann Surg 1970;172(6):946–50.
8. Barret JP, Herndon DN. Effects of burn wound excision on bacterial colonization and invasion. Plast Reconstr Surg 2003;111(2):744–50.
9. Kirn DS, Luce EA. Early excision and grafting versus conservative management of burns in the elderly. Plast Reconstr Surg 1998;102(4):1013–7.
10. Wolf SE, Kauvar DS, Wade CE, et al. Comparison between civilian burns and combat burns from Operation Iraqi Freedom and Operation Enduring Freedom. Ann Surg 2006;243(6):786–92.
11. Budny PG, Regan PJ, Roberts AH. The estimation of blood loss during burns surgery. Burns 1993;19(2):134–7.
12. Cartotto R, Musgrave MA, Beveridge M, et al. Minimizing blood loss in burn surgery. J Trauma 2000;49(6):1034–9.
13. Hart DW, Wolf SE, Beauford RB, et al. Determinants of blood loss during primary burn excision. Surgery 2001;130(2):396–402.
14. Hughes WB, DeClement FA, Hensell DO. Intradermal injection of epinephrine to decrease blood loss during split-thickness skin grafting. J Burn Care Rehabil 1996;17(3):243–5.
15. Murphy JT, Horton JW, Purdue GF, et al. Evaluation of troponin-I as an indicator of cardiac dysfunction after thermal injury. J Trauma 1998;45(4):700–4.
16. Edrich T, Friedrich AD, Eltzschig HK, et al. Ketamine for long-term sedation and analgesia of a burn patient. Anesth Analg 2004;99(3):893–5.
17. Bainbridge LC, Simmons HM, Elliot D. The use of automatic blood pressure monitors in the burned patient. Br J Plast Surg 1990;43(3):322–4.
18. Schaner PJ, Brown RL, Kirksey TD, et al. Succinylcholine-induced hyperkalemia in burned patients. 1. Anesth Analg 1969;48(5):764–70.
19. Han T, Kim H, Bae J, et al. Neuromuscular pharmacodynamics of rocuronium in patients with major burns. Anesth Analg;99(2):386-92.
20. Martyn JA, Chang Y, Goudsouzian NG, et al. Pharmacodynamics of mivacurium chloride in 13- to 18-yr-old adolescents with thermal injury. Br J Anaesth 2002;89(4):580–5.
21. Johnson KB, Egan TD, Kern SE, et al. Influence of hemorrhagic shock followed by crystalloid resuscitation on propofol: a pharmacokinetic and pharmacodynamic analysis. Anesthesiology 2004;101(3):647–59.
22. Demling RH, Ellerbe S, Jarrett F. Ketamine anesthesia for tangenital excision of burn eschar: a burn unit procedure. J Trauma 1978;18(4):269–70.
23. Hersack RA. Ketamine's psychological effects do not contraindicate its use based on a patient's occupation. Aviat Space Environ Med 1994;65(11):1041–6.
24. Lindner K, Brinkmann A, Pfenninger E, et al. Effect of vasopressin on hemodynamic variables, organ blood flow, and acid-base status in a pig model of cardiopulmonary resuscitation. Anesth Analg, 1993;77:427–35.
25. Olinger GN, Hottenrott C, Mulder DG, et al. Acute clinical hypocalcemic myocardial depression during rapid blood transfusion and postoperative hemodialysis: a preventable complication. J Thorac Cardiovasc Surg 1976;72(4):503–11.

26. Denlinger JK, Nahrwold ML, Gibbs PS, et al. Hypocalcaemia during rapid blood transfusion in anaesthetized man. Br J Anaesth 1976;48(10):995–1000.

27. Hauser CJ, Boffard K, Dutton R, et al. Results of the CONTROL trial: efficacy and safety of recombinant activated Factor VII in the management of refractory traumatic hemorrhage. J Trauma, 2010;69(3):489–500.

28. Knudson MM, Cohen MJ, Reidy R, et al. Trauma, transfusions, and use of recombinant factor VIIa: a multicenter case registry report of 380 patients from the Western Trauma Association. J Am Coll Surg 2011;212(1):87–95.

29. McHugh GJ, Norpethidine accumulation and generalized seizure during pethidine patient-controlled analgesia. Anaesth Intensive Care 1999;27(3):289-91.

30. Williams PI, Sarginson RE, Ratcliffe JM. Use of methadone in the morphine-tolerant burned paediatric patient. Br J Anaesth 1998;80(1):92–5.

31. Hettiaratchy S, Dziewulski P. ABC of burns: pathophysiology and types of burns. BMJ 2004;328(7453):1427–9 [erratum in BMJ 2004;329(7458):148].

32. Arrowsmith J, Usgaocar RP, Dickson WA. Electrical injury and the frequency of cardiac complications. Burns 1997;23(7-8):576–8.

33. Wilson CM, Fatovich DM. Do children need to be monitored after electric shocks? Journal Paediatr Child Health 1998;34(5):474–6.

34. Ducic I, Shalom A, Rising W, et al. Outcome of patients with toxic epidermal necrolysis syndrome revisited. Plast Reconstr Surg 2002;110(3):768–73.

35. Schulz JT, Sheridan RL, Ryan CM, et al. A 10-year experience with toxic epidermal necrolysis. J Burn Care Rehabil 2000;21(3):199–204.

36. Shortt R, Gomez M, Mittman N, et al. Intravenous immunoglobulin does not improve outcome in toxic epidermal necrolysis. J Burn Care Rehabil 2004;25(3):246–55.

Perioperative Nursing Considerations in Burn Care

Patricia A. Fortner, RN, MSN, MEd, CNOR

KEYWORDS

• Perioperative • Nursing care • Burns • Skin graft surgery

The American Burn Association estimates that approximately 3000 people will die every year as a result of residential fires, and another 500 will die from other burn sources including motor vehicle and aircraft crashes and contact with electricity, chemicals, or hot liquids and substances. About 55% of the estimated 45,000 US acute hospitalizations for burn injury in recent years were admitted to 125 hospitals with specialized facilities for burn care.[1]

Patients with severe burns require specialized care because of their susceptibility to infection and potential complications from inhalation injury and/or shock. Certain wound treatments and specialized operative interventions have been shown to reduce patient length of stay.[2] These treatments, including skin grafting surgeries and highly specialized wound care, are best delivered in burn centers and are important in increasing the likelihood of survival and reducing complications and adverse outcomes.[3]

Criteria for admission to a specialized burn center are as follows[4]:

- Partial-thickness burns of greater than 10% of the total body surface area (TBSA).
- Burns that involve the face, hands, feet, genitalia, perineum, or major joints.
- Third-degree burns in any age group.
- Electrical burns, including lightning injury.
- Chemical burns.
- Inhalation injury.
- Burn injury in patients with preexisting medical disorders that could complicate management, prolong recovery, or affect mortality.
- Any patient with burns and concomitant trauma (such as fractures) in which the burn injury poses the greatest risk of morbidity or mortality. In such cases, if the trauma poses the greater immediate risk, the patient's condition may be stabilized initially in a trauma center before transfer to a burn center. Physician judgment is necessary in such situations and should be in concert with the regional medical control plan and triage protocols.
- Burned children in hospitals without qualified personnel or equipment for the care of children.

United States Army Nurse Corps, CR Darnall Army Medical Center, Fort Hood, TX 76544, USA
E-mail address: pat.fortner@us.army.mil

Perioperative Nursing Clinics 7 (2012) 35–52
doi:10.1016/j.cpen.2011.12.006
1556-7931/12/$ – see front matter © 2012 Elsevier Inc. All rights reserved.

periopnursing.theclinics.com

Box 1
Characteristics of burns

First-Degree

Cause: sunburn, scald burn

Appearance: bright pink, light red

Texture: minimally edematous; blanch to touch

Surface: small blisters; dry

Sensation: painful

Second-Degree: Superficial Partial-Thickness

Cause: exposure to dilute chemicals, flash flame, very hot liquids

Appearance: bright or mottled red; possible skin discoloration over time

Texture: may blanch to touch; thickened but pliable

Surface: enlarging, weepy blisters

Sensation: painful

Second-Degree: Deep Partial-Thickness

Cause: direct contact with flame; chemical burns

Appearance: red and dry; white-yellow, mottled; considerable scar formation

Texture: moderate edema

Surface; no blister formation

Sensation: decreased sensation

Third Degree

Cause: flame, high voltage electricity, hot grease, tar, caustic, concentrated chemicals, hot metal

Appearance: waxy white, brown, or black

Texture: leathery, coarse, nonpliable,

Surface: dry

Sensation: painless

Fourth Degree

Cause: prolonged exposure to flame or high voltage electricity

Appearance: black; extends through skin, subcutaneous tissue and into underlying muscles, tendons, ligaments and bone

Texture: charred with eschar

Surface: dry

Sensation: painless

- Burn injury in patients who require special social, emotional, or rehabilitative intervention.

Specialized burn centers also treat trauma patients and those with complicated wounds or special conditions that result in the loss of skin, like toxic epidermal necrolysis, the most severe form of the exfoliating disorders, a rare but potentially lethal condition characterized by manifestation of a cutaneous drug reaction[5] and by sloughing of the skin. Burn centers also treat patients with Stevens-Johnson syndrome and erythema multiforme, milder variants of the exfoliating disorder. These patient require the skin care expertise of a specialized burn center.

Burn centers are staffed by a multidisciplinary team of burn specialty–trained, board certified general and plastic surgeons; critical care physicians; anesthesiologists; physicians in burn fellowships; physical medicine and rehabilitation physicians; nurses; physician assistants; occupational and physical therapists; respiratory therapists; dieticians; pharmacy personnel; psychological and psychiatric personnel; social workers; case managers; and chaplains. Nursing is represented by critical care nurses, wound care nurses, nurse practitioners, clinical nurse specialists, progressive care nurses, research nurses, and perioperative nurses. Burn center staff have a special commitment to the care of the burn patient.

People burn themselves in many different ways. Burns can be intentional or accidental, caused by carelessness or stupidity. Burn centers routinely care for patients injured when a candle is left burning next to drapes, someone tries to move flaming cooking oil off of a stove or leans too close to an open flame on a stove and their clothing catches fire, or the engine in a car explodes after a motor vehicle collision. Homeless people start fires to keep warm or to cook and the fire burns out of control. Turkey fryer burns occur seasonally, and burns from adding gasoline to smoldering coals in a grill is not just a summertime injury; both bring burn victims to specialized facilities.

Industrial fires bring patients to the burn centers as well. Bulldozers rupture gas lines, tanker trucks blow up, utility workers come in contact with power lines, or dry cleaning plant employees smash their hands in steaming hot clothes pressers. Toxic chemical burns are seen when employees are exposed to sulfuric, nitric, hydrochloric, and hydrofluoric acids; alkalis; gasoline; fuel; solvents; or phenol or fall into vats of tar. People drunkenly fall into campfires or the garbage they are burning, blow themselves up in methamphetamine labs, play with fireworks and sustain life-threatening injuries, or use a lit match to see into a gas can. And sadly, the tortured souls of the mentally ill self-immolate or turn a companion into a raging fireball.

Children are burned accidentally or intentionally. They may pull a pan simmering on the stove onto themselves, put their hands on a just-opened oven door, or be burned when placed in a bathtub of too-hot water. As in Afghanistan, wives and children in some villages may be punished by having boiling water or oil thrown on them.

The 2011 National Burn Repository reviewed the combined data set of acute burn admissions for the period between 2001 and 2010. Key findings included the following:

- Nearly 70% of burn patients were men. The mean age for all patients was 32 years. Children under the age of 5 accounted for 18% of burns, whereas patients age 60 or older represented 12% of injuries.
- Seventy percent of reported total burn sizes were less than 10%TBSA, and these patients had a mortality rate of 0.6%.The mortality rate for all patients was 3.9%, and it was 7.1% for fire/flame injuries.
- The two most commonly reported causes were fire/flame and scalds, which accounted for almost 8 out of 10 reported. Scald injuries were most prevalent in children under age 5, whereas fire/flame injuries dominated the remaining age categories. Seventeen percent of patients did not have a designated cause of injury.
- Sixty-eight percent of the burn injuries with known places of occurrence were reported to have occurred in the home. Sixty-five percent of patients with known circumstances of injury were identified as accident or nonwork–related.
- During the 10-year period from 2001 to 2010, the average length of stay for both female and male patients declined from roughly 11 days to 9 days. The mortality

rate decreased from 4.5% to roughly 3% for male and from 6.8% to 3.6% for female patients.

- Deaths from burn injury increased with advancing age, burn size, and presence of inhalation injury. For patients under age 60 and with a TBSA between 0.1% and 19.9%, the presence of inhalation injury increased the likelihood of death by 20 times.
- Pneumonia was the most frequent clinically related complication and occurred in 5.8% of fire/flame-injured patients. The frequency of pneumonia and respiratory failure was much greater in patients with 4 days or more of mechanical ventilation than those with less than 4 days. The incidence of clinically related complications for patients with 0 days of mechanical ventilation increased with age and topped out at 20% for patients age 80 and over.
- For survivors, the average length of stay was slightly greater than approximately 1 day per percentage TBSA burned. For those who died, the total hospital stay was roughly 3 weeks for burn patients with TBSA values below 70% and decreased from 3 weeks to 1 week for the larger burn categories.
- Overall, the charges for a patient who died were over 3 times higher than for a survivor. Additionally, hospital charges per hospital day for patients who died averaged nearly $10,000 more than for patients who survived.[6]

In combat, burn injury accounts for 5% to 10% of combat casualties.[7] Individuals who are burned during combat most commonly sustain significant flame injuries along with polytrauma from injuries caused by conflict with the enemy or in military training accidents.[8] Polytrauma sustained may include significant open extremity injuries that result in amputation, open abdominal wounds, skull fractures, and traumatic brain injuries.

The severity of the burn is generally determined by the intensity of thermal injury to which the patient was exposed, the duration of exposure, and body areas affected. The depth of the injury cannot be ascertained immediately. Thermal injury results in concentric rings of varying degrees of tissue damage. A central zone of necrosis is surrounded by a zone of stasis which, depending on the adequacy of the resuscitation, can either remain viable or proceed to cell death.[9]

When determining the percentage of the burn in the field, the entire palmar surface of the patient's hand is approximately 1% of TBSA.[10] Computerized burn programs help map the patient's burns and assist in resuscitation in burn centers.

A number of factors are predictive of mortality in burn injuries. Burn size, presence or absence of inhalation injury, and extremes of age have been reported as predictive.[11] Age is an important factor because children under the age of 2 have very thin dermis and are prone to deeper burns. Around age 50, the dermis begins to lose thickness and elasticity and predisposes older people to deeper burns. The location of the burn also is a determinant of depth, because the dermis varies throughout the body. Comorbidities include obesity, heart disease, hypertension, medication, and alcohol and/or drug use. Renal failure and insufficiency are also markers for poor outcomes after burn injury.

Preoperative preparation for the individual patient often begins before a major burn victim even reaches the burn center. Notification of an impending arrival of a patient begins the process for the burn center team. Burn critical care nurses set up the intensive care unit (ICU) room and the supplies and equipment needed to begin resuscitation in the ICU. Respiratory therapists check the ventilator and organize bronchoscopy equipment. Central and arterial line kits are in close proximity.

If the patient is reported to be unstable, the crash cart may be moved to outside of the patient's assigned room. The portable x-ray machine and electrosurgery units are close. Extra staff may be recruited if the burn is large, because major burns are very labor-intensive.

Emergency personnel at the scene of the injury have likely already placed intravenous lines (IVs) and intubated the patient by the time of arrival at the nearest hospital. If the patient meets admission criteria, the burn center is contacted for transfer approval and the patient transported for appropriate specialized burn care. The burn center's dedicated flight team, an air ambulance, or, depending on distance, ground transportation, may be dispatched to pick up the victim.

Once at the burn center, initial simultaneous assessments include airway, breathing, and circulation. Assessment of the extent of the burn and fluid resuscitation is begun. Large-bore IVs, central lines, and arterial lines are placed as needed. Outside urinary catheters and IVs are replaced with temperature-monitoring Foley catheters and large-bore IVs with tubing appropriate for the burn center's pumps. Cultures are taken of the patient's wounds. Blood is sent to the laboratory for type and crossmatching and for laboratory assessment. An oral gastric tube is placed. Tetanus immunization is administered if it was not given at the local hospital.

Smoke inhalation injury occurs below the glottis and is caused by products of combustion. Bronchoscopies are performed to diagnose and treat inhalation injuries. Diagnosis requires a history of exposure to products of combustion and a bronchoscopy that reveals carbonaceous material or signs of edema or ulceration. Bronchoscopy is considered the gold standard for diagnosis of a smoke inhalation injury.[11] Mechanical ventilation is the gold standard for inhalation injuries. The preplaced endotracheal tube may be replaced with a larger size at this time.

Burn eschar is intact, avascular, necrotic dermis that results from a burn. It acts like a tourniquet as swelling begins and may generate enough interstitial pressure to impair capillary filling and cause ischemia in the acute stage of the burn injury. Deep partial- or full-thickness circumferential burns may cause compartment syndrome of the extremities, abdomen, and chest and restrict circulation and breathing. Escharotomies may be required. The most frequently occurring extremity complications due to inadequate escharotomies are amputation and sepsis.[12]

The surgeon uses electrocautery to slice through the midaxillary line on the thorax or laterally and medially on the extremities in order to relieve pressure and expose subcutaneous tissue. Escharotomy is usually performed in the first 24 to 48 hours postburn. At some facilities, escharotomy is a bedside procedure.

Fasciotomies may be required for patients who had high voltage injuries with entrance or exit wounds on one or more extremities or because compartment pressures are increasing. Fasciotomies are usually performed in the operating room (OR).

Many surgeons believe that optimal burn care requires early excision and grafting, so accurate estimation of burn depth is crucial. The depth of the burn is difficult to determine with any certainty because wound appearance changes over the first days after injury and is dependent on the type and quality of care, mechanism of injury, age of the patient, duration of exposure, and many other variables.[13] A burn appearing shallow on day 1 may appear considerably deeper by day 3. This demarcation of the burn is a consequence of thrombosis of dermal blood vessels and the death of the thermally injured skin cells. Superficial burns may convert to deeper burns because of necrosis of ischemic areas, infection, desiccation of the wound, or the use of vasoactive drugs during resuscitation from shock.[14] Donor site wounds may also convert to deeper wounds. The wisdom of the practice of early excision and grafting has been borne out in the finding that early operations decrease septic complication.[15]

When the patient is declared by the surgeon to be sufficiently resuscitated with fluids and electrolytes stabilized or when the surgeon decides the burn wound must be treated to save the patient's life, the next step is to remove the dead skin, excise the burn, and graft the remaining wound with autograft or allograft. The perioperative staff examines the schedule and the patients already posted in the immediate future, determines with the surgeon patient priorities, and plans are made for the surgical procedures.

Preparation for the patient's first and subsequent surgical interventions requires coordination of the entire burn team. Significant amounts of blood can be lost during the excision, harvesting, and grafting surgery. Blood products must be ordered, ready before the patient is brought to the OR, and kept within close proximity. The blood bank should respond quickly to requests for additional packed red blood cells, fresh frozen plasma, or platelets. Preplanning and ordering required units by the surgeons and the anesthesiologist allows the surgery to proceed.

In general, 1 cc of reconstituted whole blood is required for each square centimeter of excised wound. Therefore, if 1000 cm^2 will be excised, approximately 2 units of packed red cells and 2 units of fresh frozen plasma should be available.[16] It is not uncommon for patients with major burns undergoing the first few surgical procedures to lose large amounts of blood.

HYPOTHERMIA

One of the big concerns in caring for burn patients is the prevention of hypothermia. Burn patients have difficulty with thermoregulation and are often unable to maintain their core body temperature because of evaporative heat loss from disrupted, burned skin. The latent heat of evaporation of water is 31.5°C. Above this temperature the energy source for evaporation will come from the environment rather than the patient. If the room temperature falls below 31.5°C (temperature-corrected with room humidity), the caloric vector is reversed, and energy radiates from the patient to the environment.[17]

In the OR, major burn patients are especially at increased risk of hypothermia because large areas of the body are totally exposed, and open wounds allow evaporative heat loss during the excision and grafting of the burn wounds. Although inspired gas, IV fluids, and blood products are warmed, the patient's core body temperature can plummet rapidly.

The burn OR ambient temperature should be set at a minimum at 88°F and should be able to be adjusted to 98 to 100°F as needed (**Fig. 1**). The ability to adjust the temperature manually in the individual OR as opposed to calling a centralized system is a plus for the burn patient. Unlike regular ORs where the temperature is set for the comfort of the surgical staff and the patient can be kept warm with forced-air methods, the main focus in the burn OR is the life of the patient.

OPERATING ROOM PREPARATION

The OR must be ready when the patient is brought into the room. As the instruments and supplies needed for the scheduled procedure are readied by the surgical technician, the rest of the perioperative team checks and sets up for the patient. With a large burn, four teams, each consisting of two or three surgeons, burn fellows, residents, and medical students, may be scrubbed. Four or more electrosurgical units should be present so that each team working can achieve homeostasis as quickly as possible. In patients with large burns, an area without a burn may not be available. Many burn ORs use a Megadyne MegaSoft reusable patient return electrode pad, which lies on top of the mattress over the length of the OR bed, is covered by a sheet, and has a female port that attaches to the electrosurgical unit. The advantage to this

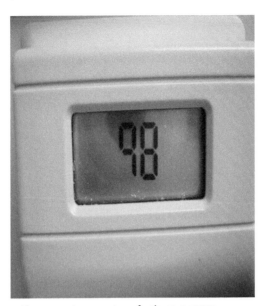

Fig. 1. Common operating room temperature for burn surgery.

grounding gel pad is that it is does not need to be in direct contact with the patient's skin. The patient merely has to be lying on top of it to be grounded.

The hydrosurgical debridement system and the gas-driven clysis machine are also made available for use during the surgery. The debridement system uses a pedal-powered high-pressure jet of sterile saline from a handpiece that cuts through the eschar, irrigates, and aspirates the wound at the same time. The pressure of the saline is controlled by a power setting on the machine. Numerous 3000-mL bags are used during a large burn procedure. Aspirated fluid is collected in large suction canisters.

The gas-driven foot pedal-operated clysis machine (called the Pitkin machine in some facilities) assists the surgeon in instilling subcutaneous lactated Ringer IV solution mixed with 1 mL epinephrine 1:100,000 into the planned split-thickness donor sites. Clysis of fluid under the donor site decreases bleeding by increasing tissue pressure (**Fig. 2**). The injected solution also creates a flatter surface for harvesting. Spinal needles and infusion tubing with a stopcock regulate the flow of the fluid. Filled 60-mL syringes with spinal needles attached are also made available for additional use.

Tourniquet machines should be checked before the start of the procedure. A variety of sizes of disposable cuffs must be available. Suction capabilities must be tested and monitored throughout the procedure. The debridement system and the clysis machine function with fluid; much of it would end up on the floor if suction were inadequate.

Custom-made packs are most cost beneficial in a burn OR. These packs can be built to the facility's specifications and revised as needed. Major burn packs should have multiple drapes, electrocautery pencils, suction tubing, a large number of staplers and numerous laparotomy and burn sponges, various types of disposable blades, and dressings commonly used.

A variety of knives are used for debridement and excision of the burn wound. Goulian (Weck) knives have a handle on which a blade is inserted, and a guard is placed over the blade. Guards range from 4/1000 to 16/1000 of an inch and regulate

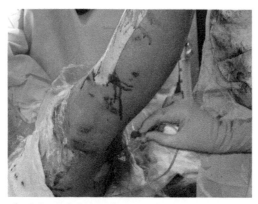

Fig. 2. Introduction of subdermal clysis to harvest site.

the depth of the debridement or excision. The Goulian knife is used for smaller or more delicate areas like the lower arms, hands, and face.

A Blair or Watson knife is much larger, with an adjustable guard. A 6-inch blade is inserted into the handle. The Blair knife is used to excise huge pieces of burned skin on the trunk and limbs. Multiple Weck and Blair blades are included in many burn centers' surgical packs because the blades become dull quickly and need to be replaced often during a large burn procedure.

The gas-powered dermatome is used most often to harvest skin for grafting (**Fig. 3**). It uses disposable blades and has various plates, 1 to 4 inches in width. The thickness of the graft to be taken is adjustable. A skin mesher is another invaluable tool in the burn OR Harvested skin is spread on a disposable plastic Dermacarrier board. The surgical technician passes the skin on the plastic dermacarrier over a cutting roller by ratcheting the handle back and forth. The harvested skin must be kept moistened while waiting to be used.

The back table should be set up in the same way for every patient so that relief personnel have little or no difficulty locating items quickly. An electric fluid warming basin is sterilely draped and turned on, and the perioperative nurse adds liters of

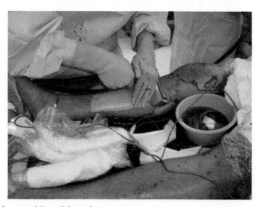

Fig. 3. Harvesting donor skin with a dermatone.

normal saline with 10 mL of epinephrine 1:100,000 per liter to begin warming. Burn sponges (laparotomy sponges without the radiopaque tie) are layered with Telfa, rolled, and then soaked in the epinephrine-saline solution. (Telfa prevents the sponge from sticking to the wound.) These "epi laps" are used over the donor sites and excised skin to help deter bleeding. Thrombin is also added to the sterile field and is drawn up in 10-mL syringes with a sprayer tip attached. Thrombin is used as an aid to hemostasis on donor and excision sites whenever oozing blood or minor bleeding from capillaries and small venules occurs.

Double- or triple-staffing is often a necessity because of the high temperature of the OR during a major burn procedure and in order to keep up with the rapid pace and the needs of three to four teams of surgeons. Those personnel working in the sterile field may rotate out at intervals to cool off, shower, change scrubs, and get a drink or nourishment. The perioperative nurse, in addition to other required duties, should be observant of the surgical team, especially those inexperienced in the burn OR. The burn OR is a high-stress environment; wearing heavy fluid-resistant gowns, face shields, and double gloves adds to the stress of the unaccustomed. Frequently they become overheated and must be assisted from the room.

PREOPERATIVE ASSESSMENT

Burn intensive care patients' families are frequently at the patient's bedside or in the family waiting room before surgery for the first few procedures, but family of patients who have prolonged hospitalizations and multiple surgical procedures usually are not present before surgery as their family member's time in the hospital lengthens. When there are relatives present, the perioperative nurse communicates with them to assure them that their family member will be cared for to the best of the burn center's ability. It is unwise, as with any preoperative assessment, to tell the family that "everything will be fine."

Much of the preoperative assessment is obtained from the electronic chart (medical history, previous surgeries to include those associated with this burn admission, allergies, and so forth), and from the patient's nurse at the bedside. These critical care burn nursing experts spend 8 to 12 hours a day for many days, weeks, and sometimes months caring for their patients and know almost everything about them. This preoperative assessment allows the perioperative team to plan for the patient's care in the OR. Verification of the patient's information begins at the bedside. The surgeon, the patient's critical care nurse, anesthesia personnel, and the perioperative nurse identify the patient with a two-patient identifier, the procedure to be performed per the operative consent, and they sign the verification paperwork before the patient is taken to the OR.

ADMISSION TO THE OR

Anesthesia and the OR and staff must be completely set up and ready before the transfer process begins. With a large burn, the patient is accompanied from the burn intensive care unit by a number of personnel to include the anesthesia provider, respiratory therapy personnel, and several critical care nurses.

The first position of the patient determines where the patient is prepared for induction of anesthesia. Patients to be prone are prepared on their ICU bed. Once the patient enters the OR, the anesthesia staff commands the organization of the immediate patient care. No action is taken with the patient until the anesthesia providers give the OK. Electrocardiogram leads are placed on the back and, in a large burn, are usually stapled to the patient's skin (the patient's wound will be wet, and the leads do not stick). The pulse oximeter is applied to whatever area is accessible and is often prepped into the sterile field as are the Foley tubing and central lines. Femoral lines are also reenforced with staples.

Once anesthesia is induced and the provider gives the go-ahead, the perioperative team descends on the patient. If the patient is to be in the prone position, the cervical spine is stabilized, IV lines and Foley catheter are protected, and he or she is log-rolled over onto perioperative staff's open arms and positioned on gel chest rolls, pillows, and foam padding. Care is taken with genitals, large abdomens, and pendulous breasts. Properly positioning a morbidly obese patient takes a team effort, and several labor-intensive moves may be required to align the patient on the operating bed correctly. After the patient is positioned, the wet dressings are quickly cut off and removed. When the dressings are off, the perioperative team at the surgeon's direction begins to remove the hundreds of staples that are holding previously placed temporary grafts in position. Once the staples are removed, the patient is prepped. Large burns usually require a total body prep in order to make all potential donor sites available for harvesting. Additional personnel are required to hold the patient's extremities or roll the patient slightly laterally in order to perform a good surgical skin prep. Ceiling hooks and IV poles can also help hold an extremity for prepping.

Chlorhexidine gluconate diluted with normal saline is the solution used for burn wounds in most burn centers. The burn wounds are not scrubbed with the prep solution; the solution is "sopped" on. Chlorhexidine gluconate should not be used on the face or head because of the possibility of damage to the eyes. Betadine should be used instead.

After the patient is draped and the team is ready to begin the procedure, a final time out is called. The surgeon, anesthesia provider, perioperative nurse, and surgical technician verify that the required instruments, supplies, and equipment are present in the room; sites are marked as appropriate; and that the patient and the procedure are correct. A two-patient identifier is used.

Because many major burn patients are unable to wear a hospital identification band because of their burns and because of frequent dressing changes, patients' identification is affixed to the end of their ICU bed. The perioperative nurse removes the identification band from the end of the bed, completes the verification process with the team, and replaces it.

SURGICAL INTERVENTION

The back table, Mayo instrument stand, and other required equipment are positioned; electrosurgical, debridement, and clysis machines are plugged in and started; suction tubing is attached; and the surgical procedures begin. There are two types of procedures to debride burn wounds. The tangential excision removes the nonviable tissue (eschar) with a thin slicing motion until punctate bleeding is observed. Tangential excision can be accomplished with a dermatome, an electrocautery device (**Fig. 4**), and a Weck (**Fig. 5**), Blair (**Fig. 6**), or regular knife blade. Tangential excision can result in copious blood loss. Active bleeders are cauterized, and thrombin is sprayed on the wound. When the wound is completely excised, it is dressed in Telfa and epinephrine-saline soaked burn laparotomy sponges. Extremities are wrapped with elastic bandages to decrease oozing. Pressure is applied to areas that cannot be wrapped. Surgeons then move on to excise additional burn sites in preparation for grafting. It has been observed that large-volume blood and blood product replacement is associated with increased mortality in adult burns.[18]

Fascial excision is the complete excision of all skin and subcutaneous tissue down to the muscle fascia layer. Experienced surgeons can perform this type of excision quickly using the electrocautery device.[13] This excision is indicated when underlying subcutaneous tissues are burned and should be considered in life-threatening, invasive wound

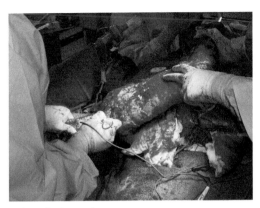

Fig. 4. Burn excision using electrocautery.

sepsis, especially when fungal organisms are involved.[12] The technique does lead to contour defects, which can be cosmetically displeasing to the patient.

Coverage of the patient's wound after excision can be accomplished in several ways. The most beneficial is the autograft. An autograft is tissue transplanted from one part of the body to another part of the body.

A split-thickness skin graft includes the epidermis and part of the dermis. Its thickness depends on the donor site and the requirements of the patient. Split-thickness autograft is harvested by a dermatome (see **Fig. 3**), a gas-driven instrument that slices thin layers of skin from the patient for use in grafting. The thickness of the graft can be selected on the dermatome, and the width is determined by the size of the blade used. The donor site may be reharvested if needed after healing.

The thighs, abdomen, and buttocks are the preferred donor sites, because the skin is thicker. Split-thickness grafts are frequently used in burn care because they can cover large areas and the rate of autorejection is low. Split-thickness grafts are either meshed to allow greater coverage of the burn wound or used as sheet grafts, that is, the donor skin harvested is placed directly on the excised burn wound (**Fig. 7**).

Sheet grafts are commonly used on the hands and face because they are more cosmetically pleasing for the patient. Sheet graft is not meshed but may be perforated

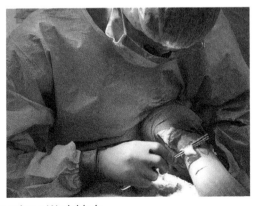

Fig. 5. Burn excision using a Weck blade.

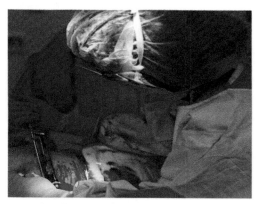

Fig. 6. Excising burn wound with a Blair blade.

(pie-crusted) with a knife blade during the procedure or postoperatively to allow the release of accumulated fluid.

Full-thickness skin grafts are used mainly in reconstructive procedures. A full-thickness skin graft consists of the epidermis and the entire thickness of the dermis. The donor site is either sutured closed directly or covered by a split-thickness skin graft.

After the donor skin is harvested, it is passed off to the surgical technician (see **Fig. 8**), who then carefully spreads it evenly on a dermacarrier. The surgeon informs the technician at which skin ratio to mesh the harvested skin. The surgical technician places the proper cutting roller (1.5:1, 2:1, 3:1, and 4:1 [most commonly used]) into the mesher and passes the dermacarrier through the mesher with the ratchet handle (**Fig. 9**). Multiple pieces of meshed skin may be required during the harvesting and grafting portion of the surgery, and even the experienced surgical technician is kept busy. Unmeshed skin is kept in a labeled bowl of saline. Meshed skin on carriers awaiting grafting is kept moist with saline.

If the general condition of the patient does not allow for harvesting of his or her own skin (because the patient is too sick), the surgeon does not want to create another wound to be healed, or the patient does not have sufficient unburned skin for grafting,

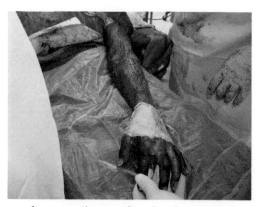

Fig. 7. Split thickness graft on arm, sheet graft on hand.

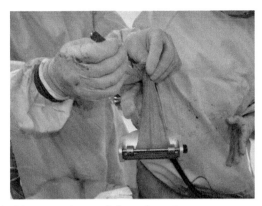

Fig. 8. Surgical technician removing graft from dermatone.

allograft may be used as a temporary covering. Allograft (or homograft) is split-thickness human cadaver skin that is supplied frozen in varying lengths from a tissue bank. This skin is used to cover large, excised burn wounds until the patient can grow his or her own skin or until a permanent skin substitute is used. Allograft is considered a temporary biological dressing.

Allograft

- will adhere and increase vascularization on a prepared wound bed;
- will decrease loss of fluids, proteins, and electrolytes and drying of the recipient bed;
- decreases bacterial contamination, diminishes pain, improves patients' ability to participate in therapy;
- is a marker of the ability of the wound to accept an autograft; and
- promotes wound healing in partial-thickness wounds.[14]

Some burn centers use xenograft (heterograft) for temporary burn wound coverage. Xenograft is tissue taken from one species and grafted to another species. Porcine dermis (pig skin) is the most commonly used xenograft. It adheres more poorly than allograft and does not undergo revascularization by the patient's body. It is used for temporary coverage of a partial-thickness burn.

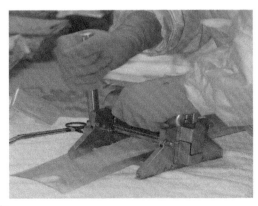

Fig. 9. Meshing skin.

The surgeons may afix the graft to the skin with staples, suture, or fibrin sealants. With a large burn it is not unusual to use more than 50 wide staplers to attach the grafts to the patient's excised wounds. Suture may be used for hands and face. Fibrin sealant, a tissue adhesive that contains protein, fibrinogen, and thrombin, is also used.

When the surgeon has completed the skin excision and grafting on the posterior of the patient, he or she may want to continue on the anterior side of the patient. The burn center should have an additional bed or a stretcher to use for turning the patient over. When the first procedure is completed and wounds are dressed, the extra stretcher is positioned next to the OR bed. Perioperative staff position themselves around the patient. When the Foley catheter and lines are protected, the anesthesia provider counts down and personnel on one side of the patient roll (flip) the patient onto the stretcher on a sheet-covered patient roller transfer device.

Staff on the opposite side quickly pull the gel rolls and other positioning devices off of the bed and remove the top layer of linens from the double-sheeted OR bed. When anesthesia personnel give the go-ahead, the patient is rolled back over to the OR bed and positioned for the anterior portion of the procedure. The patient is then prepped and draped, and the surgical intervention continues.

Wound coverage becomes a problem when the extent of the full-thickness burns exceeds the area of available donor sites. A variety of biological dressings (temporary skin substitutes) and skin substitutes have been used to overcome such wound-to-donor disproportion and to provide temporary coverage of the burns until the donor sites can be reharvested.[9]

TEMPORARY SKIN SUBSTITUTES

Biobrane is a biosynthetic wound dressing constructed of a silicone film with a nylon fabric embedded into the film that has been coated with porcine collagen. The dressing is ultrathin, semipermeable, adheres to the wound surface, is impermeable to bacteria, and controls evaporative water loss. Biobrane is supplied in sheets of film of varying sizes and as gloves. This film provides the patient with increased flexibility because of its flexibility. It is used for superficial to mid-partial-thickness burns debrided of nonviable tissue, excised burn wounds with or without meshed autografts, and donor sites.

TransCyte is a cultured temporary skin substitute. It is composed of Biobrane and newborn human fibroblasts. It is coated with porcine dermal collagen and bonded to a polymer membrane (silicone). TransCyte is transparent and allows direct visual monitoring of the wound bed. TransCyte is indicated for use as a temporary wound covering for surgically excised full-thickness and deep partial-thickness thermal burn wounds.

PERMANENT SKIN SUBSTITUTES

Integra is a bilayer, dermal equivalent matrix made of bovine collagen and glycosaminoglycan chondroitin and a semipermeable silicone layer. Some surgeons mesh Integra before applying it over the clean wound bed. After several weeks it vascularizes, the silicone membrane is peeled away, and a split-thickness skin graft is placed over the Integra. Bringing the patient back to the OR for another procedure is a drawback of Integra.

AlloDerm is a cellular dermal substitute that is obtained from cryopreserved human cadaver skin. It must be covered by a split-thickness skin graft at the time of placement. Because it is treated to remove all cells, allogenic properties are removed so it does not induce rejection. Both grafts vascularize, forming a dermal layer and an epidermal layer in one procedure.

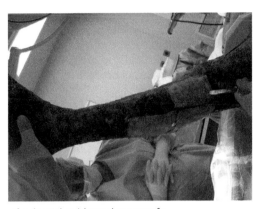

Fig. 10. Application of cultured epidermal autograft.

Cultured epidermal autograft is used to provide permanent coverage over large burn wounds and to replace the epidermal layer of skin on severely burned patients (**Fig. 10**). The patient's skin cells are grown from a postage stamp–sized biopsy of an unburned specimen of the patient's skin. The cells in the epidermis are separated and grown in a tissue culture on a layer of irradiated mouse cells for approximately 3 weeks. The cells multiply to form sheets of skin ranging from 2 to 8 cell layers thick. Cultured epidermal autograft is very fragile.

Dressings, topical antimicrobials, wound vacs (negative-pressure wound therapy, described later), immobilization for the grafted areas, and the donor sites are selected case by case, procedure by procedure by the surgeon. Topical antimicrobial agents limit fungal growth and colonization of burn wounds.

Silver sulfadiazine is a topical sulfonamide/silver antibacterial agent used as a topical burn cream on burns, including chemical burns. It prevents the growth of a wide array of bacteria, as well as yeast, on the damaged skin. It is supplied in a 1% cream or aqueous suspension. The patient may experience pain, burning, or itching after application. The treated area may appear blue-gray. Silver sulfadiazine must be wiped off of the burned skin surface, which may cause additional discomfort and pain for the patient.

Mafenide acetate 85 mg/gm (Sulfamylon) cream, applied topically, produces a marked reduction in the bacterial population present in the avascular tissues of second- and third-degree burns. It is used in the treatment of gram-negative and gram-positive organisms, including *Pseudomonas aeruginosa* and certain strains of anaerobes. Mafenide acetate is supplied in rolls, sheets, and gloves. Mafenide acetate 5% powder is also available to be mixed in the OR or at the bedside for the soaking of dressings. Soaked burn laps are layered over the grafted areas, covered with woven gauze, and elastic or woven net bandages are rolled over the extremity as pressure dressings to minimize dead space under the graft, protect the graft from sheering, and allow the antimicrobial agent to reach the wound.

Silver nitrate 0.5% is a broad-spectrum antimicrobial agent used in the treatment of second- and third-degree burns. It does not penetrate burn eschar and needs bulky and frequent dressing changes, which limits its use. Silver nitrate is diluted with sterile water, which can lead to electrolyte imbalance. It permanently stains everything it touches a brown-black color.

Dakin solution is diluted sodium hypochlorite solution and is used in the treatment of gram-positive and gram-negative bacteria in burn patients. It is also effective in the treatment of viruses, molds, fungi, and yeast and is effectively used for odor control.

Bacitracin is a nontoxic, water soluble topical antibiotic used chiefly against gram-positive organisms of burn wounds but not against gram-negative organisms or fungi. It is used often on face burns.

The chest, abdomen, and back are often dressed with the topical antimicrobial agent chosen by the surgeon, solution-soaked burn laps, and a large burn dressing sponge that covers the areas. The surgical technician staples elastic surgical net to each side of the large burn sponge, and after it is placed on the patient, the net is stretched and stapled together. This procedure allows the wet dressings to stay in position as the ICU staff turn and move the patient. This process is repeated for the back wound, and the two are stapled together.

Donor sites may be dressed with fine mesh gauze and scarlet red, a bismuth and petroleum gauze, or a silver-impregnated wound barrier dressing. For outpatients with small burn wounds and small harvest sites, anesthesia personnel may inject a local anesthetic for pain relief.

Negative-pressure wound therapy uses a sealed wound dressing connected to a vacuum pump. The continued vacuum draws out fluid from the wound and increases blood flow to the area and assists in healing. The foam dressing is cut to the size of the wound, and then a sticky film drape is placed over the foam to create a seal. A vacuum tube is connected through an opening in the film drape to a canister on the side of a vacuum pump.

Tracheostomies are indicated because prolonged intubation may be associated with complications, and therefore conversion to a formal tracheotomy is usually performed for long-term management of the airway in critically ill patients.[12] Amputations may be performed on major burn wounds because of the massive burn damage to muscle and bone or because of uncontrolled infection.

When the surgical procedure is almost completed, the perioperative nurse is responsible for calling the ICU to give a report of what has occurred in the OR. Using the SBAR (situation-background-assessment-recommendation) technique, the perioperative nurse relays to the patient's nurse which procedures the patient has undergone and the sites of each procedure. The amount of IV fluids and blood products given, estimated blood loss, and urinary output are reported. Vital signs, amount of tissue excised and grafted, and type of antimicrobial agents and dressings placed are also reported. Questions from the receiving nurse are answered, and a time frame is given for arrival. In addition to obtaining information from the electronic intraoperative and anesthesia notes, the critical care nurse at the bedside also receives a preprinted drawing ("naked man") noting which grafts were placed and the specific type of graft.

When the procedure is completed the patient is transferred to the bed, taking special care to maintain lines, Foley catheter, dressings, and wound vac; covered with a foil blanket; and transferred ventilated to the ICU. In the ICU, the anesthesia provider gives a detailed report to the patient's nurse.

Patients may undergo numerous surgical procedures aimed at removing eschar and covering burn wounds with allograft to reduce the potential for bacterial growth and sepsis. Allograft may be exchanged every few days in a "sick" patient, and the perioperative staff begin to feel as if they know the patient well. Major burn patients may come back 15 to 20 or more times for surgical procedures.

The burn OR is a hot, humid, stressful, demanding environment. It is not for the delicate, easily upset, or queasy. Massive tissue debridement is discarded in large red-bag–covered biohazard boxes that fill rapidly. Wounds ooze, blood drips or squirts onto the floor, small pieces of burned skin and fat always seem to land on the floor, and oftentimes there is a repellant odor. But there is something unique about burn nursing.

All burn nurses who share this most emotionally challenging profession earned their place with lots of blood (the patient's), sweat (the perioperative staff's), and sometimes tears. The knowledgeable staff realize that their patient's survival from burn wounds is not guaranteed. It takes the entire burn center team working together to provide the best management of the burn patient.

Box 2
Terminology

Allograft: Graft from one individual to another individual of the same species; includes cadaveric, living related, and living unrelated donors. Also called homograft.

Autograft: Graft from one area of the patient's body to another area of the same patient.

Clysis: Infusion of fluid, usually subcutaneously, for therapeutic purposes.

Conversion: Progressive necrosis in the depth and width of the burn.

Debridement: Removal of loose, devitalized, necrotic tissue on the wound using mechanical or sharp technique.

Dermis: Inner layer of skin that contains blood, lymph vessels, hair follicles, and glands that produce sweat and sebum.

Desiccation: Process of drying out.

Epidermis: Outer layer of the skin made of squamous and basal cells. The deepest part of the epidermis also contains melanocytes that produce melanin, which gives the skin its color.

Eschar: Intact, avascular, necrotic dermis that results from a burn.

Escharotomy: Surgical incision through the burn eschar (necrotic skin). Eschar is not removed.

Excision: A surgical procedure requiring incision through the deep dermis, subcutaneous, and deeper tissues of open wounds, or burn eschar.

Fascial excision: Complete excision of the skin and subcutaneous tissue down to the muscle fascia layer.

Full-thickness skin graft: Contain the epidermis and the entire dermis; usually reserved for reconstructing wounds of the head, neck, hands, and areas of the genitals and breasts.

Harvest: Removal of skin tissue for use in covering burns on other parts of the body.

Meshing: Use of a smooth plastic plate, or carrier, to move the skin graft under circular notched blades, as used in the mesh dermatome. Another method does not use a carrier; instead, it uses two opposing rollers, and the skin graft is cut as the two rollers meet.

Skin Replacement: Tissue or graft that permanently replaces lost skin.

Skin Substitute: Bioengineered cells or tissues that can be used as allograft or autograft.

Split-thickness skin graft: Contain the epidermis and a variable thickness of the upper layers of dermis, leaving the remaining layers of dermis in place to heal by secondary epithelialization from the wound edges and keratinocytes within the adnexa of the deeper dermis.

Tangential excision: Process of shaving very thin layers of eschar until viable tissue is seen.

Total body surface area (TBSA): Refers to area affected by second- and third-degree burns.

Xenograft: Tissue taken from one species and grafted to another species. Porcine dermis (pig skin) is the most commonly used xenograft to provide temporary coverage.

REFERENCES

1. American Burn Association. Burn incidence and treatment in the United States: 2011 Fact Sheet. Chicago: American Burn Association; 2011.
2. Curreri PW, Luterman A, Braun DW, et al. Burn injury. Analysis of survival and hospitalization time for 937 patients. Ann Surg 1980;192:472–8.
3. Committee on Trauma. Resources for optimal care of the burn injured patient. Chicago: American College of Surgeons; 1999.
4. Guidelines for operation of burn centers. Available at: www.ameriburn.org/chap. Accessed September 15, 2011.
5. Endorf FW, Cancio LC, Gibran NS. Toxic Epidermal necrolysis clinical guidelines. J Burn Care Res 2008;29(5):706–12.
6. American Burn Association. National burn repository. Chicago: American Burn Association; 2011.
7. Cancio LC, Horvath EE, Barillo DJ, et al. Burn support for Operation Iraqi Freedom, and related operations 2003–4. J Burn Care Rehabil 2005;26:151–61.
8. Kauver DS, Wolfe SE, Wade CE, et al. Burns sustained during combat explosions in Operations Iraqi Freedom and Enduring Freedom. Burns 2006;32(7):853–7.
9. Cioffi WG Jr, Rue LW, Buescher TM, et al, A brief history and the pathophysiology of burns. In: Zajtchuk R, Jenkins DP, Bellamy RF, editors. Conventional warfare: ballistic, blast, and burn injuries. Washington, DC: Office of the Surgeon General, Department of the Army, Borden Institute; 1990. p. 337–48.
10. American Burn Association, Advance burn life support manual. Chicago: American Burn Association; 2007.
11. Dries DJ, Management of burn injuries, recent developments in resuscitation, infection control an outcomes research. Scand J Trauma Resusc Emerg Med 2009;17:14.
12. Lawton G, Dheansa B. The management of surgical burns–a surgical perspective. Curr Anaesth Crit Care 2008;19:275–81.
13. Tenenhaus M, Rennekampff, HO. Burn surgery. Clin Plast Surg 2007;34:697–715.
14. American Burn Association. Surgical management of the burn wound and use of skin substitutes, white paper. Chicago: American Burn Association; 2009.
15. Wu XW, Herndon DN, Spies M, et al. Effects of delayed wound excision and grafting in severely burned children. Arch Surg 2002;137:1049–54.
16. Wolfe SE. The major burn. In: Barret JP, Herndon DN, editors. Principles and practice of burn surgery. New York: Marcel Dekker; 2005. p. 221–49.
17. Woodson LC. Anesthesia for acute burn injuries. In: Barret JP, Herndon DN, editors. Principles and practice of burn surgery. New York: Marcel Dekker; 2005. p. 103–34.
18. Palmeri TL, Greenhalgh DG. Blood transfusions in burns: what do we do? J Burn Care Rehabil 2004:25;71–5.

Surgical Care of Thermally Injured Patients on the Battlefield

Leopoldo C. Cancio, MD

KEYWORDS

- Burns • Military personnel • Iraq War • 2003
- Perioperative care

For young adults treated in burn centers in developed nations, the lethal area 50%—that is, the burn size lethal to one-half of a given population—has almost doubled since World War II from 43% of the total body surface area (TBSA) to 75% TBSA.[1] This achievement reflects many factors, of which improvements in wound care, perioperative care, and surgical technique have figured prominently. The challenge deployed military health care providers face is how to translate these advances to the relatively austere and unforgiving environment of the combat zone.

Thermal injuries are present in 5% to 20% of combat casualties.[2–3] Thus, on the battlefield, role IIb (forward surgical teams) and role III (combat support hospitals) facilities frequently care for patients with burns.[4] Most of these patients fall into two categories: US military casualties and local national casualties. US military casualties undergo emergency treatment and preparation for aeromedical evacuation to the United States.[5–6] Local national casualties, under the rules of engagement for the current conflicts in Iraq and Afghanistan, cannot be evacuated to the United States; these patients must receive care locally. Because local resources in both theaters are limited, US field hospitals often are responsible for providing not only emergency treatment but also definitive care. Here, the author reviews the surgical care of patients with thermal injuries as it is practiced on the current battlefield. Conceptually, burn care can be divided into three distinct, albeit closely overlapping, phases: resuscitation, wound closure, and reconstruction. Operative management may be required during each of these phases.

This work was supported by the Combat Critical Care Engineering Task Area, US Army Institute of Surgical Research.

The author has nothing to disclose.

The opinions or assertions contained herein are the private views of the author and are not to be construed as official or as reflecting the views of the Department of the Army or Department of Defense. The discussion of commercial products does not constitute an endorsement.

Medical Corps, United States Army Burn Center, United States Army Institute of Surgical Research, 3698 Chambers Pass, Fort Sam Houston, TX 8234–6315, USA

E-mail address: lee.cancio@us.army.mil

Perioperative Nursing Clinics 7 (2012) 53–69

doi:10.1016/j.cpen.2011.12.002

1556-7931/12/$ – see front matter Published by Elsevier Inc.

periopnursing.theclinics.com

RESUSCITATION PHASE
Emergency Evaluation

Initial evaluation of acutely burned patients takes place in the emergency department (ED) or equivalent in the deployed hospital. Emergency evaluation and preparation for the operating room (OR) should follow a standard sequence.[7] This sequence (the "ABCs") differs importantly from those followed for patients with nonthermal trauma, reflecting differences in physiology. The main differences between burn shock and hemorrhagic shock are the *speed* of fluid loss and the *type* of fluid lost. With respect to speed, fluid loss in burn shock can be massive, but it occurs gradually over the course of approximately 48 hours. The primary cause of this process is damage to small blood vessels ("leaky capillaries"), which permit fluid to escape into the tissues, causing edema.[8] With respect to type of fluid, in burn shock a protein-rich plasma rather than blood leaves the vascular system. This loss of circulating volume is the main cause of burn shock. In burn resuscitation, caregivers strive to achieve a balance between fluid replacement to restore the circulating volume and overresuscitation, which makes edema worse and can cause complications such as compartment syndromes. Inhalation injury further complicates burn resuscitation by directly damaging the airway and by interfering with the ability of the lungs to exchange gases.[9] Finally, other injuries may occur along with—and may complicate the management of—the burns, especially in combat casualties. Thus, a thorough search for nonburn injuries is required in all combat casualties with burns. With this protocol in mind, the ABCs of burn resuscitation are as follows:

- *Airway.* Intubate all patients with symptomatic inhalation injury, with burn size greater than 40% (because of risk of edema), with significant facial injuries or swelling (**Fig. 1**), and/or with depressed level of consciousness.
- *Breathing.* Treat patients with suspected carbon monoxide toxicity with 100% oxygen. Do chest escharotomies if needed (see later discussion).
- *Circulation.* Start two large-bore intravenous catheters, through unburned or burned skin. Start lactated Ringer's (LR) solution or similar isotonic crystalloid (eg, Plasmalyte) at an initial rate of 500 mL/hr in adult (250 mL/hr in children); see later discussion under Fluid Resuscitation for fine-tuning this rate.

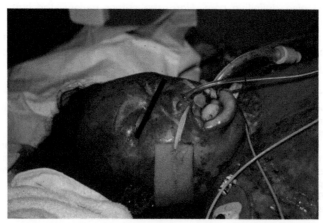

Fig. 1. Facial edema. The combination of facial burns, massive fluid resuscitation, and inhalation injury creates a high-risk scenario for airway loss. Constant attention to airway patency and, (as shown here) security, is essential.

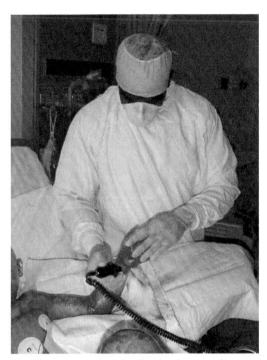

Fig. 2. Upper-extremity elevation and evaluation by Doppler flowmetry. During the burn shock phase (48 hours), the upper extremities are elevated to reduce edema and the risk of a compartment syndrome, and the pulses are checked hourly in all burned extremities.

- *Disability.* Evaluate any change in mental status, which may indicate inhalation of toxic gases or head injury.
- *Environment.* Maintain normothermia. Burn patients are at high risk for hypothermia because of impaired skin integrity. Do not cool the patient or the wounds.
- *Expose and examine.* Remove all clothing and all jewelry.
- *Extremities.* Check for peripheral pulses (radial, ulnar, dorsalis pedis, anterior tibial). Elevate burned upper extremities above the level of the heart on blankets or other objects to decrease edema and risk of compartment syndrome (**Fig. 2**).
- *Fluid resuscitation.* Measure the burn size using the rule of nines and/or a Lund-Browder burn chart (**Fig. 3**). Then calculate the initial fluid rate.
  - For adults, use the Institute of Surgical Research rule of ten[10]: LR rate = TBSA $\times$ 10. For example, for an adult man with a burn size of 60% TBSA, LR rate = 60 $\times$ 10 = 600 mL/hr.
  - For children (<40 kg), use a formula such as the Parkland formula: 24-hour fluid requirements = TBSA $\times$ weight $\times$ 4; give half of this amount in the first 8 hours. For example, for a 10-kg child with a burn size of 40% TBSA, 24-hour LR volume = (40 $\times$ 10 $\times$ 4) = 1600 mL. Give half of this amount in the first 8 hours: LR rate = 100 mL/hr. Also, give children 5% dextrose in one-half normal saline at a maintenance rate.
  - Titrate the LR rate up or down hourly to achieve the target urine output of 30 to 50 mL/hr in adults (0.5 to 1.0 mL/kg/hr in children).
  - Document the hourly ins and outs on a flow sheet (**Fig. 4**).[11]

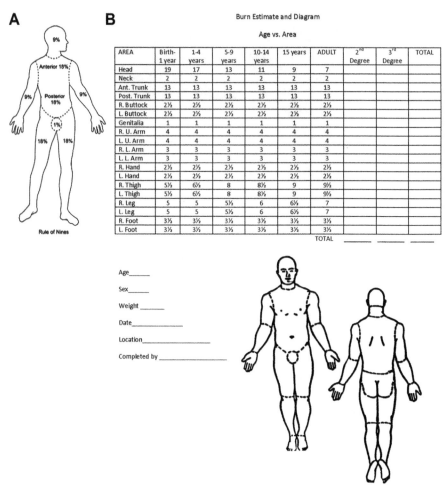

A

9%

Anterior 18%

9%   Posterior 18%   9%

(1%)

18%   18%

Rule of Nines

B

Burn Estimate and Diagram

Age vs. Area

AREA	Birth-1 year	1-4 years	5-9 years	10-14 years	15 years	ADULT	2nd Degree	3rd Degree	TOTAL
Head	19	17	13	11	9	7			
Neck	2	2	2	2	2	2			
Ant. Trunk	13	13	13	13	13	13			
Post. Trunk	13	13	13	13	13	13			
R. Buttock	2½	2½	2½	2½	2½	2½			
L. Buttock	2½	2½	2½	2½	2½	2½			
Genitalia	1	1	1	1	1	1			
R. U. Arm	4	4	4	4	4	4			
L. U. Arm	4	4	4	4	4	4			
R. L. Arm	3	3	3	3	3	3			
L. L. Arm	3	3	3	3	3	3			
R. Hand	2½	2½	2½	2½	2½	2½			
L. Hand	2½	2½	2½	2½	2½	2½			
R. Thigh	5½	6½	8	8½	9	9½			
L. Thigh	5½	6½	8	8½	9	9½			
R. Leg	5	5	5½	6	6½	7			
L. Leg	5	5	5½	6	6½	7			
R. Foot	3½	3½	3½	3½	3½	3½			
L. Foot	3½	3½	3½	3½	3½	3½			
						TOTAL	___	___	___

Age_____

Sex_____

Weight _____

Date_____

Location_____

Completed by _____

Fig. 3. (*A*) The rule of nines provides a rough first estimate of the burn size. (*B*) The Lund-Browder chart provides a more accurate estimate of the burn size.

- *Secondary survey.* Look for nonthermal trauma, which is common in combat casualties.
- *Tubes and lines.* Nasogastric tube, Foley catheter for all patients with TBSA greater than 20%. Consider arterial catheter for blood pressure monitoring and for frequent labs.
- *Prophylaxis.* Gastroduodenal ulcer (eg, proton-pump inhibitor); deep venous thrombosis (eg, low-molecular-weight heparin).

Initial Wound Care

The OR is an ideal environment for initial wound care of thermally injured patients. At the US Army Burn Center (US Institute of Surgical Research, Fort Sam Houston, TX, USA), initial wound care takes place in large shower rooms specially built for this purpose. In deployed hospitals, however, such facilities are not available. The OR provides 24-hour availability, clean-to-sterile conditions, anesthesia support,

JTTS Burn Resuscitation Flow Sheet   Page 1

Date: _____   Initial Treatment Facility: _____

Name	SSN	Pre-burn Est. Wt (kg)	%TBSA	Estimated fluid vol. pat. should receive		
				1st 8 hrs	2nd 16th hrs	Est. Total 24 hrs

Date & Time of Inury: _____   BAMC/ISR Burn Team DSN 312-429-2876

Tx Site/ Team	HR from burn	Local Time	Crystalloid (ml) Colloid	TOTAL	UOP	Base Deficit	BP	MAP (>55) / CVP	Pressors (Vasopressin 0.04 u/min)
1st									
2nd									
3rd									
4th									
5th									
6th									
7th									
8th									
Total Fluids 1st 8 hrs:									
9th									
10th									
11th									
12th									
13th									
14th									
15th									
16th									
17th									
18th									
19th									
20th									
21st									
22nd									
23rd									
24th									
24 hr Total Fluids:									

Fig. 4. US military Joint Theater Trauma System burn resuscitation flow sheet. A document such as this one should be filled out hourly during the burn shock phase. (*From* Ennis JL, Chung KK, Renz EM, et al. Joint Theater Trauma System implementation of burn resuscitation guidelines improves outcomes in severely burned military casualties. J Trauma 2008;64[2 Suppl]:S146–51; with permission.)

supplies, and manpower. Thus, the practice for burn patients on the battlefield is to initiate resuscitation in the ED as described previously, then to proceed to the OR for wound care. This care includes thorough debridement of all burn wounds using chlorhexidine gluconate and gauze. This debridement is aggressive and is intended to remove all nonviable blister tissue, debris, and foreign material. Pain control and

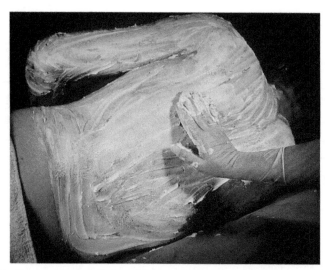

Fig. 5. Application of topical antimicrobial burn cream to burns. Note that a thick layer of an antimicrobial burn cream (like frosting a cake) is applied to the burn wound after thorough daily cleansing.

anxiety management are very important during this and subsequent painful procedures (see later discussion).

Wounds are then dressed in an antimicrobial material (**Fig. 5**).[12] There are three classes of topical antimicrobials, the most commonly used being topical silver. Since 1968, the leading source of topical silver for burn wound care has been silver sulfadiazine cream (Silvadene). Silver sulfadiazine cream has the advantage of providing silver in a slow-release formulation but requires dressing changes, wound cleansing, and replacement once or twice daily. Clean wounds of limited extent may, alternatively, be treated with silver-impregnated dressings such as Silverlon, Acticoat, or SelectSilver. These dressings also release the silver slowly and need to be changed only once every 3 to 5 days as long as the wound surface remains devoid of bacterial colonization.

The second class of topical agent is mafenide acetate (Sulfamylon). Mafenide is a highly effective topical antimicrobial agent with outstanding efficacy against gram-negative organisms, which are the leading cause of lethal burn wound infection in untreated patients. Mafenide acetate is available as a 5% aqueous solution or as an 11% cream. For care of the burn wound, the cream is ideal. The aqueous solution is most commonly used as a topical agent after skin grafting.

The third option for topical care of the burn wound is a synthetic temporary skin substitute such as Biobrane. This product is a bilaminar material whose two layers are designed to mimic the dermis and the epidermis. The dermal part consists of polyethylene mesh impregnated with collagen. The epidermal part consists of silicone with intermittent perforations to allow fluid to escape. Biobrane is an excellent choice for meticulously sterile partial-thickness burns. This material may remain in place until healing takes place underneath, at which point it will gradually separate. It requires careful daily attention and immediate removal if pus develops underneath.

When applying a burn cream—either silver sulfadiazine or mafenide acetate—it is essential to apply it as a layer, opaquely covering the entire wound. The best analogy for this application is that it is like frosting a cake. After application of a topical antimicrobial cream or material, the author most commonly places a thick gauze dressing. Coarse mesh roller gauze (eg, Kerlix) is ideal for burned extremities, but it should be applied or cut away such that continued monitoring of peripheral pulses is possible (see later discussion). Large burn dressings are useful for the torso. The face is rarely dressed. Surgical netting of various sizes is very useful to hold dressings in place.

Escharotomies and Fasciotomies

Eschar means burned skin. There are two conditions in which an urgent incision into the eschar, or escharotomy, may be needed: thoracic eschar syndrome and extremity eschar syndrome. In both cases the inelastic eschar, in combination with soft tissue edema, squeezes the underlying tissues. Escharotomy may be done with a scalpel and/or electrocautery. The key is to incise through the full thickness of the skin and into the subcutaneous fat to permit the cut edges of the eschar to retract fully. An incision that fully exposes the investing fascia is not normally required.

Thoracic eschar syndrome refers to the straightjacket-like effect exerted by circumferential deep burns of the chest. This syndrome restricts chest wall motion and respiration and may cause cardiac arrest. The treatment is chest escharotomy as an emergent bedside procedure. With chest escharotomy, normal chest excursions should immediately return.

Circumferential burns of the extremities are a major cause of morbidity following thermal injury. The author refers to the tourniquet-like effect exerted by circumferential extremity burns as the extremity eschar syndrome. This syndrome is most frequently caused by full-thickness burns that fully encompass an extremity, but it can occur in deep partial-thickness burns or in burns that do not completely encircle the limb. Beneath the tight, inelastic eschar, soft tissue edema further constricts blood flow. This constriction leads ultimately to arterial inflow obstruction, nerve and muscle damage, and limb loss. Escharotomy involves a longitudinal incision through the burned skin along the midmedial (and/or midlateral) joint lines (**Fig. 6**). The indication for the operation is the loss or progressive diminution of distal arterial flow (radial, ulnar, palmar arch in the upper extremity; dorsalis pedis or posterior tibial in the lower extremity) as measured by Doppler flowmetry. Postoperative care includes resumption of topical antimicrobials, attention to missed bleeders, and (most important) continued vigilance for distal arterial flow.

A common mistake in the care of burned extremities relates to confusion between extremity eschar syndrome and extremity compartment syndrome. In the former, the cause of constriction is the burned skin, and the operation is escharotomy. In the latter, the cause of constriction is the investing muscular fascia, and the operation is fasciotomy. Fasciotomy is not a benign procedure in a burn patient, because it opens up the deep muscles to bacterial proliferation. Thus, the author does not perform prophylactic fasciotomies in burn patients. But extremity compartment syndrome does occur in burn patients, especially when resuscitation volumes are high, when other trauma has occurred, and/or when escharotomies were delayed or inadequate. Thus, the author advocates close monitoring of burn patients, with measurement of intracompartmental pressures whenever confusion exists about the diagnosis. When performing a fasciotomy, the team must be exquisitely aware of the need to completely release all compartments in a given area. This caveat is necessitated by the fact that inadequately released or missed compartments were a fairly common finding in a recent battlefield study.[13]

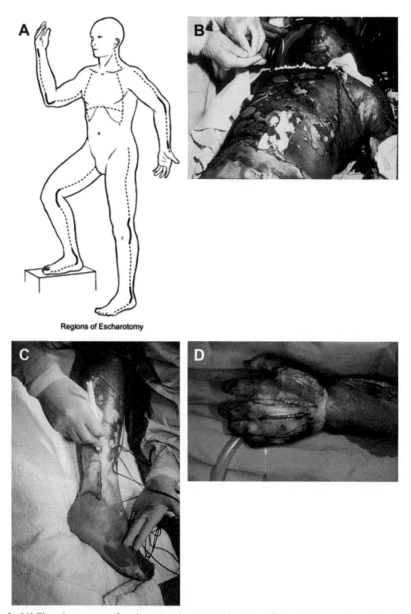

Fig. 6. (*A*) The placement of escharotomies. Note location of the incisions along the midmedial and midlateral joint lines of the extremities and in the chest area. (*From* Cancio LC, Thomas SJ. Burns [thermal, scald or chemical]. In: Farr WD, editor. Special Operations Forces medical handbook. 2nd edition. Washington [DC]: US Government Printing Office; 2008. p. 7.17–17.27.) (*B*) Chest escharotomies. (*C*) Lower extremity escharotomies. (*D*) Hand escharotomies.

WOUND CLOSURE PHASE

Fluid resuscitation is typically complete by about 48 hours postburn. At this point the surgeon must decide whether or not to perform excision and grafting: definitive removal of the burn wound and replacement of the skin with grafts. This decision is influenced by both logistical and surgical considerations. Because this procedure is resource-intensive and ties the patient to the hospital for 7 to 10 days postoperatively, it is universally discouraged for US casualties on the battlefield. Rather, US casualties are evacuated as soon as they are hemodynamically stable back to the US Army Burn Center for definitive surgical care and rehabilitation. By contrast, no such option exists for local national patients at deployed US hospitals. For these patients, the author recommends prompt excision of all full-thickness burns and those deep partial-thickness burns judged too deep to heal within 14 to 21 days postburn. Of course, there is a subjective aspect to this assessment of burn wound depth.

Local nationals with extensive burns may present in delayed fashion several days after injury. In the absence of adequate topical antimicrobial therapy, these patients may present with invasive gram-negative burn wound infection. These infections are characterized by discolored wounds and clinical evidence of sepsis. Care consists of aggressive resuscitation in the ED and intensive care unit, application of topical mafenide acetate cream (11% Sulfamylon cream), and urgent excision to fascia. Depending on the overall condition of the patient and on the appearance of the wound bed after excision, it may be reasonable to autograft at the same operation, or it may be preferable to place the wound in a topical antimicrobial agent such as 5% Sulfamylon solution overnight.

Operative Plan

Before undertaking excision and grafting, a detailed operative plan should be formulated and discussed with all members of the team. This plan should include a supply and equipment list. At a minimum, the author recommends that the following checklist be reviewed as a team before this operation:

- *Warm environment of care.* Because burn patients lose heat rapidly, intraoperative hypothermia is a major concern and must be prevented by maintaining a hot OR. For many personnel this is the most onerous aspect of burn operative care. Thus, OR temperature needs to be thoroughly discussed ahead of time.
- *Hemostatic strategy.* Burn surgery is typically bloody. A well-thought-out strategy to reduce blood loss is particularly important in the deployed hospital. The essential elements of this strategy include the following:
  - Liberal use of tourniquets for excision of the extremities, with Esmarch bandages for exsanguination.
  - Epinephrine solutions (carefully labeled) in LR solution:
    - Topical solution: epinephrine in normal saline or LR solution (1:100,000; ie, 10 mL of epinephrine 1:1000 in 1 L).
    - Subdermal clysis solution: epinephrine in LR solution (1:1,000,000).
  - Limited extent and duration of excision. For the relatively inexperienced team, this means no more than 10% TBSA excision at a single operation.
  - Bovie electrocautery.
  - Availability (in the OR at the start of the case) of typed and cross-matched packed red blood cells and fresh frozen plasma.
- *Surgical tools.* Although experienced operators may be able to make do with substandard equipment, at a minimum the following tools are needed for successful grafting:

○ Hand dermatomes for excising burns, with disposables.
○ Power dermatome for harvesting skin, with disposables.
○ Skin mesher, preferably for skin 4 inches in width with tools to mesh at ratios 1:1, 1:1.5, and 1:2.
- *Dressings and other disposables.* Burn surgery typically requires a plentiful supply of various dressings:
  ○ Laparotomy sponges for use during hemostasis.
  ○ Coarse-mesh roller gauze (eg, Kerlix).
  ○ Rolls of 3% bismuth tribromophenate in petrolatum on fine-mesh gauze (Xeroform) for donor sites and grafted sites.
  ○ Elastic bandages (Ace) for extremity hemostasis.
  ○ Staplers for affixing skin grafts.
  ○ Surgical netting of various diameters for securing gauze dressings.

Surgical Technique

Following induction of general anesthesia, all of the wounds are undressed and the patient undergoes sterile preparation of all of the burn wounds with chlorhexidine gluconate solution. Then the areas to be grafted and the donor sites are widely draped. A Zimmer dermatome (most commonly electrically powered in the deployed setting) is used to harvest skin at a depth of 8 to 12/1000 inch. The most commonly used donor sites are the anterior and lateral surfaces of the thighs. However, any body part may serve as a donor site. Special donor site considerations include the following: The scalp should undergo clysis with a solution of 1:1,000,000 of epinephrine in LR solution by using a 60-mL syringe and an 18-gauge needle. This procedure is essential for hemostasis in the scalp, which otherwise will bleed profusely. In other areas, clysis may be done to facilitate donor site harvesting from irregularly contoured areas such as the ribs (**Fig. 7**). After harvesting, hemostasis of the donor site is facilitated, if needed, by temporary application of a laparotomy sponge soaked in the

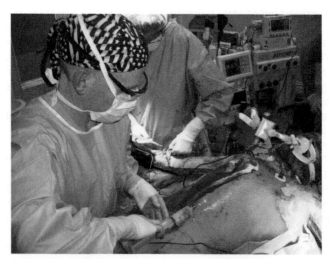

Fig. 7. Subdermal clysis. A solution of epinephrine (1:1,000,000) is injected beneath the skin to permit donor site harvesting from a difficult area; in this case, the left anterior abdomen. Skin has already been harvested from the right anterior abdomen. Meanwhile, another operator excises the right upper extremity.

topical epinephrine solution. Then Xeroform gauze is stapled in place. A coarse mesh gauze dressing may then be applied, followed by surgical netting or an elastic bandage.

Autografts may be meshed or left unmeshed. Most often the author applies unmeshed skin to functional areas such as the face and hands. It is reasonable to apply skin meshed 1:1.5 or 1:2 to other areas. Skin meshed at higher ratios such as 1:3 or 1:4 take a long time to heal, during which time the exposed wound bed in the interstices is vulnerable to desiccation, necrosis, and infection. Thus, the author rarely applies skin meshed this widely without an overlying layer of cadaver allograft skin, which is not available on the current battlefield.

Excision of the wound is the most important part of the operation. Burn wounds may be excised to fascia or tangentially. Fascial excision is reserved for extensive, deep, full-thickness burns. Examples of wounds that merit fascial excision include those that are infected and those that extend into the fat. This level of excision results in a better skin graft success rate ("take rate") than does excision to fat, but it results in a less optimal functional and cosmetic outcome. Tangential excision is preferred for partial-thickness wounds and for clean full-thickness burns of limited extent.

The technique of fascial excision includes use of Bovie electrocautery, scalpel, and/or curved Mayo scissors to excise the entire thickness of the skin and subcutaneous tissue off the investing fascia (**Fig. 8**). Tangential excision, by contrast, involves the use of a large hand dermatome such as a Brown, Humby, Braithwaite, or similar instrument for large areas and a small tool such as a Goulian knife (Weck, Inc) for detailed work, for example, on the hands (**Fig. 9**).

The end point of tangential excision is viable tissue. When the wound is partial-thickness, the deep dermis is alive and well perfused and the end point of excision is the presence of punctuate microvascular bleeding. When, however, the wound is full-thickness, the entire dermis is dead and the end point of excision is viable-appearing, well-perfused fat. When an extremity is excised under tourniquet after exsanguination with an Esmarch bandage, blood loss should be decreased, but punctate bleeding is no longer available as an end point. Rather, viable-appearing

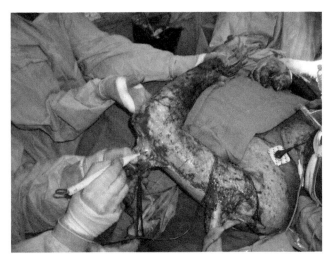

Fig. 8. Excision to fascia of deep full-thickness burns of the left upper extremity. Note previously performed escharotomies of the hand.

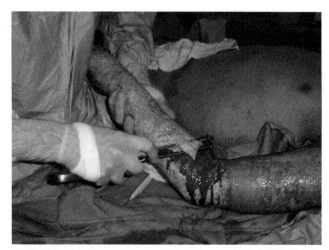

Fig. 9. Tangential excision of full-thickness burns of the left upper extremity. In this case, the level of excision is to viable fat. Note the fast rate of blood loss. The team must be prepared to complete the excision rapidly and to stop the bleeding effectively.

tissue and the absence of hemosiderin staining in the tissue are the end points. (Hemosiderin, a hemoglobin breakdown product, appears in damaged tissue as tiny dark spots. Its presence means that microvascular damage, and thus microvascular bleeding into the tissues, occurred at the time of burn.).

Excision can be bloody. Blood loss during fascial excision is achieved by careful ligation of vessels as they are encountered. Blood loss during tangential excision without a tourniquet in place may be achieved by working rapidly and immediately after excision by applying laparotomy sponges soaked with topical epinephrine solution and compressive dressings. Recombinant human thrombin spray (eg, Recothrom) may be applied to the wound to assist with hemostasis before dressing application. Following about 5 minutes of compression, hemostasis is completed using electrocautery. A square inch at a time, the laparotomy sponges are eased off the wound bed, small squirts of irrigation fluid are delivered with a Toomey syringe to help clear the field of clots, and electrocautery is performed. Blood loss during excision with a tourniquet in place may merely be delayed. However, application of laparotomy sponges and elastic bandages to the extremity before the tourniquet is let down is essential.

Once hemostasis is obtained, the wound is reinspected to ensure adequacy of the excision's depth. The operation will be unsuccessful if the grafts are placed onto nonviable tissue. Reexcision of areas is preferred to such an outcome. Next, skin grafts are affixed to the viable wound bed using either staples or sutures (**Fig. 10**). Staples are easier to use but require time and pain control postoperatively at the time of removal. Sutures are preferable for smaller wounds in children.

There are several options for postoperative dressings. At the US Army Burn Center, the author commonly applies either silver nylon dressings followed by gauze moistened with sterile water or wound veil (Dermanet Wound Contact Layer) followed by gauze soaked in 5% Sulfamylon solution. An excellent alternative that seems to speed engraftment is a negative-pressure wound therapy device such as vacuum-assisted closure (VAC). In the deployed setting, the author most commonly has used Xeroform gauze in combination with VAC (**Fig. 11**).

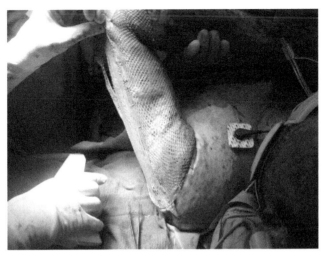

Fig. 10. Placement of meshed skin grafts. Use of skin staples helps speed the operation.

Immobilization of skin grafts is an important component of postoperative care. Immobilization may be achieved with a VAC, with a plaster or thermoplastic splint, and/or with surgical netting. Effective immobilization is particularly important when the graft crosses a joint.

Rarely is it wise to leave an excised wound bed ungrafted. These large open areas are prone to desiccation, tissue death, and infection, even with optimal local wound care. In US burn centers, if the wound bed is of questionable viability and/or if the risk of autograft loss is judged to be high, cadaver allograft may be

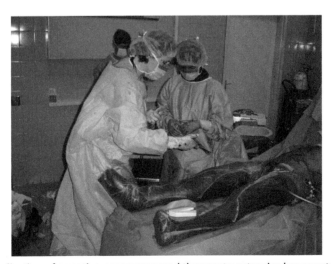

Fig. 11. Application of negative-pressure wound therapy to extensive lower-extremity graft sites. Application of negative-pressure wound therapy dressings like these is time-consuming, but these dressings seem to speed and enhance graft take.

used instead of autograft. This temporary biologic dressing protects the wound while helping to prepare it for ultimate autografting. Unfortunately, this option is not available on the battlefield. On rare occasions, the author has used a close relative (mother or father) as a donor of fresh allograft for pediatric patients with extensive burns. A negative-pressure wound therapy (VAC) dressing also helps prepare the wound. In all other cases, immediate closure with autograft should be performed.

Postoperative Wound Care

Skin graft sites remain dressed for 3 to 5 days postoperatively, at which time they are inspected and redressed every day or two until the grafts are fully engrafted and the interstices (mesh holes) are filled in with new cells. Then, a gentle topical ointment such as bacitracin or Aquaphor (Eucerin) should be applied daily. Gentle range-of-motion exercises should begin after the first dressing change. Staples should be removed beginning day 5 to 7 postoperatively.

Donor sites should be uncovered down to the Xeroform gauze directly on the wound on postoperative day 1. Xeroform remains in place until healing occurs underneath. Then the gauze gradually separates from the wound and should be trimmed. During healing, donor site dressings should gradually dry out and should remain well adherent. Nonadherent donor site dressings with underlying purulence indicate possible infection and may signal the need for dressing removal and application of a topical antimicrobial agent. Donor sites may also develop cellulitis, manifested by surrounding erythema and, possibly, systemic signs of infection.

Excision of Special Areas

The most challenging body part from the standpoint of excision and grafting is the hand. In patients with massive burns, excision of the hand is probably best postponed until the majority of the rest of the body has been excised. This delay permits more time to be devoted to the hands, with care not to injure tendons or joints. In contrast to the rest of the body, in the case of the hand, it may be preferable to err on the side of tissue preservation rather than on the side of overzealous excision. Palmar surfaces are rarely excised acutely because they often heal spontaneously, albeit with contractures. Obviously, necrotic fingers are best treated by acute amputation. Exposed tendons mandate an aggressive approach to preservation including, wherever possible, immediate coverage with autograft or allograft. The services of an orthopedic or plastic hand surgeon may be critical in these patients.

It is unusual to excise and graft the face in acute burn care. The depth of facial skin, the presence of numerous hair follicles, and the vascularity of the tissue cause the face to have excellent healing characteristics. Deep full-thickness burns of the face may need to be grafted, in which case thick, unmeshed skin should be applied according to the concept of facial aesthetic units.

Postoperative Care

Patients undergoing a major excision and grafting operation may emerge from the OR cold, coagulopathic, and acidotic. Preventing such instability by proactive intraoperative management and timely completion of surgery requires experience and foresight. Nevertheless, postoperative resuscitation may be required. The author often prepares a combination of 1 ampule (50 mEq) of sodium bicarbonate and 100 mL of

25% albumin in 1 L of Plasma-Lyte crystalloid solution for rapid postoperative infusion when difficulty is anticipated. The key to postoperative resuscitation is to understand the patient's physiologic status. Early postburn (during the first 48 hours after injury) patients with burns of 20% or more of the TBSA are likely to require ongoing resuscitation for burn shock, as described previously. During subsequent weeks, patients may emerge from the OR with an intravascular volume deficit from intraoperative hemorrhage, which may be massive; loss of one entire blood volume during an extensive excision is not uncommon. These patients may not have received enough blood products in the OR and may need transfusion of packed red blood cells and fresh frozen plasma analogous to mechanical trauma patients. The care of these patients may also be complicated by septic shock, because large (>40% TBSA) contaminated burn wounds typically release bacteria into the bloodstream when excised.[14] Such patients are likely to require ongoing support with fluids, pressors, and antibiotics. Close attention to the dressings and to the hematocrit is important in order to detect and correct any postoperative bleeding.

Pain Management

Management of pain and anxiety is critical throughout a burn patient's course, from resuscitation through rehabilitation. Nevertheless, pain control in burn patients is typically inadequate.[15] During the resuscitation phase, the cornerstone of pain management is frequent small doses of an intravenous narcotic such as morphine or fentanyl. Later, burn patients rapidly become habituated to standard doses of narcotics, and a more potent narcotic such as hydromorphone (Dilaudid) may be more convenient. In addition, methadone may be useful for background pain treatment. Intravenous ketamine is a near-ideal drug for painful procedures in these patients[16] for the following reasons: (1) the dose can be titrated from analgesia through general anesthesia, (2) airway reflexes are maintained, (3) emergence phenomena are easily prevented by concomitant use of a benzodiazepine, and (4) in contrast to narcotics and other general anesthetics, ketamine supports the blood pressure in all but the most severely catecholamine-depleted patients. Because burn patients experience painful procedures on a daily basis for weeks to months, they come to dread these procedures and develop anticipatory anxiety. This anxiety can be managed by oral or intravenous lorazepam (Ativan) medication before the procedure is begun.

RECONSTRUCTION PHASE

Reconstruction is a major component of burn care of local nationals in the deployed setting, because many of these patients present after wounds have healed, usually without adequate initial surgical or rehabilitative care. Such deficits in early care predispose to formation of contractures that can severely limit function or, in the case of extrinsic ectropion of the eyelid, pose a high risk of blindness. Therefore, the author recommends that the deploying surgical team be familiar with the following operations:

- Release of burn scar contractures involving the major joints (especially neck, axilla, elbows, and knees).
- Ectropion release of the upper and lower eyelids.
- Palmar scar release.
- Web space scar contracture release.

SUMMARY

Care of burn patients is physically demanding, psychologically stressful, and logistically costly.[4] At the same time it can be immensely rewarding. Recognizing these challenges and developing a plan to meet them is, in the author's experience, an essential component of effective team leadership on the battlefield. In the OR, the major physical stressor is heat, which, nevertheless, is essential to prevent hypothermia in these patients with impaired skin integrity. The sources of psychological stress are manifold. First, a salient feature of the personal experiences of many surgeons, nurses, and other personnel during the current conflicts is lack of prior experience in burn care. Second, thermal injury is associated with a significant mortality; such mortality accrues despite weeks of effort. The rewards may also be difficult to appreciate, likewise accruing only after weeks of labor. Third, providers may believe that definitive care of local nationals falls outside of the deployed hospital mission, despite the requirements of the Geneva Convention. Fourth, the care of burned local nationals exposes the providers to difficult cultural factors, which may include child and domestic abuse, acts of terrorism, and uncertainty in the face of inadequate long-term follow-up.

Given that successful burn care requires the concerted efforts of a multidisciplinary team, leaders must exert themselves to build such a team and to strengthen morale if burn care in the deployed setting is to be successful. And yet, the author's experience has repeatedly been that such team building is in fact possible. The author believes, for example, that demonstrating a successful outcome after an otherwise devastating injury to a local national is a morale booster on the battlefield. This success represents not an individual but a team accomplishment.

REFERENCES

1. Pruitt BA Jr. Combat casualty care and surgical progress. Ann Surg 2006;243(6): 715–29.
2. Pruitt BA, Goodwin CW, Mason AD Jr. Epidemiological, demographic, and outcome characteristics of burn injury. In: Herndon DN, editor. Total burn care. London: WB Saunders; 2002. p. 16–30.
3. Emergency war surgery. 3rd United States revision. Washington (DC): The Borden Institute; 2004.
4. Stout LR, Jezior JR, Melton LP, et al. Wartime burn care in Iraq: 28th Combat Support Hospital, 2003. Mil Med 2007;172(11):1148–53.
5. Renz EM, Cancio LC, Barillo DJ, et al. Long range transport of war-related burn casualties. J Trauma 2008;64(2 Suppl):S136–44.
6. Cancio LC, Horvath EE, Barillo DJ, et al. Burn support for Operation Iraqi Freedom and related operations, 2003 to 2004. J Burn Care Rehabil 2005;26(2):151–61.
7. Advanced burn life support course instructor's manual. Chicago: American Burn Association; 2001.
8. Pham TN, Cancio LC, Gibran NS. American Burn Association practice guidelines burn shock resuscitation. J Burn Care Res 2008;29(1):257–66.
9. Cancio LC. Airway management and smoke inhalation injury in the burn patient. Clin Plast Surg 2009;36:555–67.
10. Chung KK, Salinas J, Renz EM, et al. Simple derivation of the initial fluid rate for the resuscitation of severely burned adult combat casualties: in silico validation of the rule of 10. J Trauma 2010;69(Suppl 1):S49–54.

11. Ennis JL, Chung KK, Renz EM, et al. Joint Theater Trauma System implementation of burn resuscitation guidelines improves outcomes in severely burned military casualties. J Trauma 2008;64(2 Suppl):S146–51.

12. Cancio LC, Howard PA, McManus AT, et al. Burn wound infections. In: Holzheimer RG, Mannic JA, editors. Surgical treatment— evidence-based and problem-oriented. New York: W. Zuckschwerdt Verlag GmbH; 2001. p. 671–83.

13. Ritenour AE, Dorlac WC, Fang R, et al. Complications after fasciotomy revision and delayed compartment release in combat patients. J Trauma 2008;64(2 Suppl):S153–61.

14. Mozingo DW, McManus AT, Kim SH, et al. Incidence of bacteremia after burn wound manipulation in the early postburn period. J Trauma 1997;42(6):1006–10.

15. Patterson DR, Tininenko J, Ptacek JT. Pain during burn hospitalization predicts long-term outcome. J Burn Care Res 2006;27(5):719–26.

16. Owens VF, Palmieri TL, Comroe CM, et al. Ketamine: a safe and effective agent for painful procedures in the pediatric burn patient. J Burn Care Res 2006;27(2):211–6.

A Burn Intensive Care Unit Nurse's Perspective

Andrew Wallace Jr, RN, ASN

KEYWORDS

- Burn care • Nursing • Intensive care • Perioperative care

For burn patients, the day of surgery can come as quickly as hours or as late as days, possibly even weeks, after the initial injury. With reconstructive and scar revision procedures the patient's surgical journey may not end until years after the burn. It is the first few surgical procedures that concern the burn intensive care unit (BICU) nursing staff the most. After a large burn encompassing 30% total body surface area or greater, the first excision and grafting (E&G) procedures are the most critical. Experienced burn surgeons and BICU staff know that there is no substitute for early, aggressive excision of the burn wound in patients with large burns.

Deep or Full thickness burns produce an inflammatory response where the eschar (the deep cutaneous necrotic tissue produced by thermal burn or corrosive application) and the viable tissue meet. This area is where bacterial growth in the eschar attracts polymorphonuclear leukocytes (neutrophils) that release large amounts of proteolytic enzymes and inflammatory mediators.[1] As a result, these mediators start separating eschar from the granulating tissue that produces nonsurgical burn scars. These untreated burns result in limited mobility and disfiguring scars. By removing the burned and devitalized tissue, burn surgeons are able to save the patient's life as well as improve appearance and function.

Research shows that E&G surgical intervention not only improves survival rates, it decreases the length of hospital stay and decreases the total cost associated with burns.[1] Additionally, it has been shown that mortality decreases even in the presence of inhalational injuries. Early surgical removal of the burn wound and covering of the surgical site with autograft or allograft became the standard of practice in 1976.[1] The presence of a burn wound, partial- or full-thickness, is a constant drain on the patient's reserves; surgical intervention and closure of the burn wound significantly limit this drain.

The main objective in burn care is closure of the wound with the patient's own epidermis. Sometimes closure is spontaneous, but often surgery is required to

The opinions or assertions contained herein are the private views of the author and are not to be construed as official or as reflecting the views of the Department of the Army or the Department of Defense.

United States Army Institute of Surgical Research, Fort Sam, Houston, TX 78234, USA

E-mail address: andrew.wallacejr@amedd.army.mil

Perioperative Nursing Clinics 7 (2012) 71–75
doi:10.1016/j.cpen.2011.12.005
1556-7931/12/$ – see front matter Published by Elsevier Inc.

remove the eschar and cover the wound with autologous skin graft or autograft (harvested from the patient). When there is not enough autograft to cover the wound, the gold standard is use of allograft, or cadaver skin, to cover the wound.[1] If fresh skin is available, it may take as a skin transplant until the body rejects it, which may take weeks to months. This temporary covering allows donor sites to heal before they are reharvested.

The burn patient is transported to the operating room (OR) in a manner different from the way other patients go in. The patient is brought in on the specialty bed (Kin Air bed or Fluid Air bed, KCI, San Antonio, TX, USA) that he or she was on in the BICU. A thermoreflective blanket covers the patient to maintain and help prevent any heat loss while moving from the warm environment of the BICU out into the cooler hallway. Hemodynamic monitoring continues throughout the transport process until the patient is connected to the monitors in the OR. All pumps are transported along with his or her vasoactive drugs, and intravenous (IV) fluids are kept running during the transport to the OR and during the procedure. Up to three IV poles with two three-chamber pumps each are transported with the patient. Additional staff are required to help maneuver the bed, the monitors, and the IV poles for a safe and quick trip to the OR.

Respiratory therapists are part of the transport team because the volumetric diffusive respirator ventilator is often used in the OR. The respiratory therapist wears a backpack harness containing a green fiberglass oxygen tank that is connected to the ventilator, which remains connected to the patient during the transport.

The entire OR staff waits, wearing protective gowns, masks, eyewear, and gloves, as the patient is rolled into the room. Once lines are secured the team is ready to move the patient over to the OR table to position, prep, and drape appropriately for the beginning of the E&G procedure.

Positioning the burn patient prone for any part of the surgical procedure has its own set of issues. Whenever the patient is turned onto a prone position for harvesting of grafts or debridement of burns, the potential exists for invasive lines to be dislodged, Foley catheter, trauma, and, most critical, unintentional extubation, which would cause decompensation and require emergent return to the BICU. Additionally, pronating a patient often results in facial and scleral edema, even with the use of special face padding and goggles.

Burn wounds have been classified into three categories: first-, second- and third-degree. The burn community prefers to use the terms *superficial* or *partial-thickness* and *full-thickness* to describe burn injuries. Typically, a first-degree burn is not considered part of the burn wound because it involves only the epidermis and heals quickly with the growth of new keratinocytes.[1] The second-degree, or partial-thickness, burn destroys all of the epidermis as well as portions of the dermis. Some partial-thickness burns heal without surgical intervention if the follicular bulge area is uninjured. It is thought that stem cells originating from the bulge area produce the new keratinocytes that repopulate the epidermal basal cell layer including sebaceous glands and hair follicles within the new epidermis.[1] This burn wound is extremely painful, making cleaning and debridement a horrific procedure for the patient and a stressful daily activity for the burn nurse. Partial-thickness burns that can be left alone are treated with topical antimicrobial agents.

A tangential excision is used on a partial thickness burn by removing thin layers of burned skin until the surgeon reaches viable dermis or the subcutaneous fat is exposed. Several instruments may be used to excise the burn wound including knives with adjustable guards that allow the surgeon to vary the depth of penetration or dermatomes. The Rosenberg knife, Goulian knife, Watson knife, and, VersaJet water dissector are some examples of tangential excision instruments used in burn procedures. With a tangential excision, healthy tissue is determined by the presence of dermal or subcutaneous bleeding.[2] The burn is debrided to a shiny white dermal surface with fine copious blood flow.

Deep-, or full-thickness, burns involve the entire thickness of the dermis and extend into the subcutaneous fat. If small enough, a full-thickness burn wound will heal as the eschar separates and granulation occurs, but this process leads to hypertrophic scars. Surgical intervention is most likely the only choice in any full-thickness burn injury. This leather-like injury is relativity painless and nonblanching. All other burned areas have pain associated in and around the burn wound. Early E&G decreases the pain associated with the burn wound over time.[2]

Current practice is to excise as much of the burn wound as possible during the initial surgical procedure, taking into account the stability of the patient.[1] The excision of the burn wound can be a tangential excision that removes the burned tissue, leaving as much of the underlying viable tissue as possible. With this type of excision body contours are better preserved, hospital stay is decreased, reconstructive surgical procedures are fewer, and patients report less associated pain.[1]

The fascial excision is a formal integumentectomy excision that removes the subcutaneous fat including the lymphatic tissue down to the fascia. Although less blood loss is expected, this procedure creates what is known as "step-offs." During a fascial excision, the surrounding viable tissue and underlying fat result in an uneven surface that creates the step-off. Typically, electric cautery can be used to excise the burn wound, decreasing bleeding as the tissue is removed.

Meshed split-thickness autograft gives a less desirable cosmetic appearance but is required when available donor sites are limited or the patient has suffered an extensive burn. The meshed skin is achieved by running the sheet graft through the surgical mesher at a determined ratio of expansion (1:1 through 4:1). The parallel slits created in the sheet graft allow the skin to be expanded when being placed on the excised wound bed. The newly placed meshed autograft will begin to reepithelialize across the interstices connecting the meshed skin to provide wound closure. Time to closure is dependent on the patient and ratio of expansion. When healed, the graft retains the wafflelike meshed appearance, texture, and color. Meshed graft is protected by the surgical dressing for 3 to 5 days, allowing the graft to adhere to the wound bed. Leaving the dressings on for such an extended time allows the fibrin seal that initially holds the autograft in place to advance with capillary growth and collagen production.[2] Allograft may be placed over the larger expanded autograft to protect against shearing. The use of negative-pressure dressings or Wound Vacs (KCI, San Antonio, TX, USA) may also be used to cover and protect the newly placed autograft, keeping the dressing in place for the same 3 to 5 days postoperatively.

Each type of graft placed on the patient has specific implications in the postoperative period for the BICU staff. Split-thickness sheet autograft, or sheet graft, is a continuous layer of donor skin that is harvested from the donor site and secured to the patient with staples, sutures, or adhesive strips. This type of graft is usually reserved for cosmetic areas like the face, neck, hands, and fingers. The thickness of the graft harvested typically is 0.009 to 0.020 inches as determined by the burn surgeon to maximize outcome for the individual patient. The thicker grafts tend to shrink less and provide a better cosmetic appearance.[2] With sheet grafts, typically 12 to 24 hours post graft placement the nurse and surgeon evaluate the graft and remove any blood clots and accumulated serum. The sheet graft must be assessed and evaluated frequently to remove any subgraft hematoma or seroma by needle aspiration or by placing a small incision to roll out fluid or clots. Rolling out the seroma toward the edge of the graft with a cotton-tip applicator during the first several days can become an hourly task.

Burn patients typically become hypothermic while in the OR despite increased room temperature (85°–95° F) and draping while on the OR table. It is not uncommon for the BICU room temperature to be increased to between 85° and 100° F. Most nurses choose to have the room as warm as possible because they understand that postoperative hypothermia increases the risk of vasoconstriction, hypoperfusion, and metabolic acidosis. Heat lamps and space blankets along with increased room temperature are efficient ways to warm the patient and provide an optimal environment for graft take. Another piece of equipment that should be available is a rapid infuser with heating capabilities. This device allows for a fast delivery of IV fluids for hypovolemic shock and gives the staff another option to reverse the hypothermic state the patient may return in.

For postoperative patients deemed at risk for hemodynamic insufficiency, the US Army Burn Center prepares vasopressin, norepinephrine, and dobutamine prior to the patient's return from surgery. The first drug of choice is vasopressin. In the Army BICU, vasopressin is hung as a first line drug in hemorrhagic shock associated with excessive blood lose related to extensive E&G. Vasopressin acts on the renal system by increasing the water permeability of the distal tubules and collecting ducts, allowing water reabsorption. It also acts on the cardiovascular system by increasing peripheral vascular resistance and in turn increasing the arterial blood pressure. Vasopressin is an on/off drug; there is no need to titrate up or down. The standard dose is 0.04 U/min or 2.4 U/h.

If the patient continues to require cardiovascular support, norepinephrine is the next choice in the bedside arsenal. Norepinephrine acts on both α_1-and α_2-adrenergic receptors, causing vasoconstriction and increased peripheral vascular resistance. At increased doses and when combined with other vasopressors it can lead to limb ischemia. In causing vasoconstriction and limb ischemia, norepinephrine is basically starving the newly placed graft of blood flow and increasing the risk of poor or no graft take and ultimately risking another surgical procedure for the patient to undergo. For this reason norepinephrine is not considered as a first line vasopressor in the Burn ICU. Norepinephrine is hung and titrated up, down, and off very quickly, if possible.

Since Dobutamine is a direct-acting agent whose primary activity results from the stimulation of the β_1-adrenoceptors of the heart which increases contractility and cardiac output, it is of little use immediately postoperatively because the patient often has hypovolemic shock. Once fluid and blood products have restored intravascular volume, dobutamine may be used.

At the Army Burn Center, having two "bricks" at the bedside is a practice used for a large-burn patient returning from the OR. The brick is a consolidation of elements used during a massive transfusion into one bag and is only used in the face of ongoing bleeding and severe hypotension while waiting for blood products. The brick is composed of 100 mL of 25% albumin and 1 A of sodium bicarbonate in 1 L Ringer lactate. If the mean arterial pressure is low (<50), the physician may transfuse the patient postoperatively with packed red blood cells, plasma, and/or platelets.

The hypovolemic state brought on by massive blood loss in the OR and possible continued blood loss from open wounds and donor sites continues to assault the patient's hemodynamic stability. At this time, BICU nurses hang the brick while waiting for additional blood products to arrive.

Total fluids infused include colloids, crystalloids, blood products, and hypodermal clysis (subcutaneous fluid instillation). Colloids (albumin and plasma proteins) are used to increase intravascular volume; crystalloids (lactated Ringer and normal saline) help in the vascular volume but also replace the extracellular fluid. The amount of packed red blood cells given in the burn OR is a good indicator of blood loss and allows the BICU nurse to anticipate the need for more products to have on hand in the BICU.

In the burn OR, hypodermal clysis is a subcutaneous injection of saline into the dermis that allows for easier harvesting over irregular surfaces like the ribs or back. At the Army Burn Center, a solution of 1 L of Ringer lactate with 1 cc of epinephrine 1:100,000 U infused with an 18-gauge spinal needle and a pressure pump is used. This derma-infused solution is eventually absorbed into the patient's vasculature over the course of several hours. Physicians and BICU staff must be made aware of this volume to adjust the IV volume being administered and reduce the risk of fluid overload.

It is impossible to accurately estimate blood loss during burn surgery. During the procedure, blood is not collected in canisters where it can be measured but is under the patient, in surgical drapes, absorbed in sponges and towels, on the floor, and even washed down drains. The estimated blood loss is an art form established over countless surgical procedures and is a well-educated guess by the experienced burn anesthesiologist. Urine output is also a component of fluid loss and should be included in the OR to BICU report.

Donor site care is different from burn wound care; each burn facility has its own way of dressing and managing donor sites. One is Xeroform gauze stapled over the wound, Telfa and epi-laps (sterile burn sponges soaked in a solution of 10 cc epinephrine 1:100,000 U in 1 L sterile normal saline irrigation) then compressed with an elastic bandage. The dressing is removed 24 hours postoperatively. Heat lamps are applied if additional drying is required. Lamps are placed 18 to 24 in above the site for 20 minutes each hour to facilitate drying. A positioning device that elevates the limb and allows air flow around the donor site to aid in drying is effective. Some biological dressings are used, but if fluid accumulates under the dressing it can lead to infection and possible conversion to a full-thickness wound. Infection and possible conversion occurs when a donor site has decreased perfusion and the wound fluid is left to create an overly moist wound bed.

A trip to the burn OR increases the workload of the BICU, but a well-prepared nurse can receive the patient from the OR in any condition and lead the nursing team through a potentially chaotic, intense, and emergent postoperative period.

Burn care requires constant communication and attention to detail; it is a physical form of nursing that requires mental and physical toughness. From the warm environment and long hours at the bedside caring for the patient to the interaction with the families, burn nurses are at the front of patient care. With the proper education and training, those who choose the rewarding title of burn nurse make a difference every day in the lives of their patients and their patients' families.

REFERENCES

1. Herndon DN. Total burn care. 3rd edition. Philadelphia: Elsevier; 2007. Chapters 11, 13, 14, 15.
2. Carrougher GJ. Burn care and therapy. St Louis (MO): Mosby; 1998. Chapter 10.

Hope for Recovering Burn Patients—The Multidisciplinary Approach (Ultrarapid Opioid Detoxification Under Anesthesia)

Bonnie A. Jackson, RN, MSN, CCNS-C, Mary Sueltenfuss, RN, BSN, NLC, Christopher V. Maani, MD, MC, US Army*

KEYWORDS
- Burn care • Ultrarapid opioid detoxification under anesthesia
- Nursing care • Pain management

The importance of assessing pain as the sixth vital sign is well-ingrained in today's medical profession as well as in our daily practice. Treating pain, however, can open a Pandora's box with its own challenges for some patients such as burn patients, who present with a multiplicity of challenges. Consider the combat soldier who sustains extensive burns as a result of battlefield conflicts.

In addition to the initial painful insult, burn patients must endure countless wound debridement procedures, dressing changes, and multiple surgeries, which in many cases can morph the acute pain into unrelenting chronic pain. Currently, medications that act on μ-opioid receptors have proven to provide the best pharmacologic management for the relief of chronic burn-related pain. As a result, opioid analgesia has risen to the forefront of the health care professional's arsenal for the treatment of burn pain. However, prolonged opioid therapy can leave a recovering burn patient to deal with opioid dependence or addiction.[1–3]

The lack of pain education, especially in the understanding of opioid dependence and/or addiction, has been an obstacle for health care workers. Traditionally, nurses and physicians have struggled with the dilemma of evaluating when to medicate a

Disclosures: No financial disclosures.

The opinions expressed herein are those of the authors and are not to be construed as official or as reflecting the views of the US Department of Defense or the US Army.

Department of Anesthesiology, United States Army Institute of Surgical Research and Army Burn Center, Brooke Army Medical Center, 3400 Rawley East Chambers Avenue, Fort Sam Houston, TX 78234, USA

* Corresponding author.

E-mail address: Christopher.Maani@us.army.mil

burn patient's pain and when to withhold pain medication based on their perceptions of the quality and intensity of pain. Placed in this difficult position, it is understandable that some health care providers could become skeptical of or even cynical about pain that is not understood or discerned. However, it is vital that all health care providers remember that the extent and quality of pain that a patient feels can only be determined by the patient; the one who feels and experiences it. Burn-injured patients can present with intense and agonizing pain and anecdotally describe their burn pain as "excruciating" and "the worst pain that could ever be experienced." Therefore, when a patient with chronic burn pain asks for pain medication, the first question that we should ask ourselves is not whether or not we should administer the requested pain medication, but rather, in good conscience can we withhold pain medications? It is arguable that to withhold pain medications when requested by the burn patient under duress is unreasonable, even unethical.

Health care providers need to be aware that the prolonged use of opioid analgesia over an extended period of time for chronic pain control can for some patients blossom into an increased tolerance, which results in use of extremely large doses of pain medication and polypharmacy to manage their pain.[1,2] This increased tolerance is particularly true for patients with chronic burn pain. Burn patients who exhibit physical dependence or addiction often develop tolerance from their escalating doses needed to control their pain.

The distinction between opioid dependence and addiction is pivotal for both the patient and the health care provider to grasp, because there is a stigma attached to the individual that can be either self-imposed or society-branded. If patients' perceived pain prevents them from living a quality life, using a medication that helps them to have a quality life should not be labeled drug abuse.[2]

Some patients who have found themselves living in a perpetual fog, unable to function or return to the level that they and/or their family long for, reach out for help and express a desire to "get off meds." One combat veteran who sustained extensive burn injuries described himself as being "preoccupied with just living without pain and scared to miss a pain pill because of fear that the pain would return." Another patient described his daily ritual of having to continuously self-medicate to relieve his pain as a "continuous frustration." Patients may make the outcry to their care provider asking, "Is this going to go on forever? I want to start living again and get on with my life!" These patients often exhibit depression and express feelings of hopelessness at their situation. Statements such as, "I feel totally helpless, and I can't take needing that pill just to keep going from minute to minute. . ." are not unusual from this unique population. It is important that all nurses, doctors, physical therapists, counselors, social workers, and clergy be in tune to these types of comments and statements. A consult referral for the burn center's anesthesiologist to evaluate the patient and his or her medical/pharmaceutical status in the pain clinic should be initiated.[4]

During the pain clinic consultation, the burn center's anesthesiologist will thoroughly review the patient's medical, surgical, and pharmaceutical history. If traditional weaning of opioids has been unsuccessfully tried, the anesthesiologist will evaluate the patient as a potential candidate for ultrarapid opioid detoxification under anesthesia (URODA), which is available for the authors' recovering military post burn patients.[4] URODA is designed to help the patient who wants to decrease pain medication usage by reversing dependence or addiction to narcotics.[5-6]

During the anesthesia consult, patients often describe the untoward and unwelcome side effects they have experienced: respiratory depression, myoclonus, nausea, urinary retention, constipation, vomiting, itching, and/or somnolence.[2-3] Through an organized and systems-based approach, the anesthesiologist assesses the severity of burn-related pain. Questions are posed to elicit the patient's perception of the pain, emotional state, somatic preoccupation, functional status, and general perception of quality of life. The patient's responses are both acknowledged and respected. Some patients report that their burn-related pain has stopped them from participating in activities with family and friends. URODA has proven to be a viable option for some of these patients.[4]

The URODA multidisciplinary team at the authors' burn center developed a detailed and stringent URODA protocol to analyze the effectiveness of this detoxification process to achieve successful opioid detoxification and minimize patients' narcotic demands. Careful detail is given to behavioral/mental health evaluation of prospective candidates to determine if the prospective patient would be a viable candidate for the URODA procedure. A patient's self-esteem can suffer as a result of the physical effects of the burn injury, disfigurement, physical challenges, and opioid dependence and/or addiction. A patient may report, for example, that "people respect me less because they see me popping pills all day long. . .as many as 20 to 30 a day!"

In addition to medically and pharmacologically screening for prospective URODA procedure participation, the patient's psychological and support system needs are addressed by behavioral health professionals. In the authors' burn center it was agreed that refusal to follow through with a behavioral medicine evaluation or consultations would render a candidate ineligible for study participation and would be listed as exclusion criteria. American Society of Anesthesiology physical classification III or greater as well as exceeding the age of 65 years old were also exclusionary criteria.[4]

When identified as qualifying URODA, patients and their identified support person or caretaker were provided with detailed information about the URODA process by the burn center anesthesiologist with ample time for question-and-answer sessions as well as time to consider granting consent for the URODA procedure. Patients and their families were provided with contact numbers and a detailed schedule including admission date and time and explanation of events that would occur upon intensive care unit (ICU) admission.

The URODA process is well-orchestrated. Respiratory therapy, pharmacy, and the nursing staff support were coordinated; supplies, intravenous (IV) drips, and man-power were readied. Upon the patient's ICU admission, the burn center anesthesiologist administered both Versed and propofol and performed tracheal intubation with respiratory therapy personnel standing by. It was the authors' center's protocol to place the patient on a Draeger ventilator and maintain on continuous positive airway pressure mode. The patient usually remains intubated for a minimum of 24 hours while the anesthesiologist continually monitors the patient's progress and labs and orders IV drip titrations; in essence, the anesthesiologist is the URODA team quarterback and provides total oversight, ensuring the integrity of the protocol. The nursing staff titrates the drips and maintenance IV fluids and monitors the patient's response by keeping a continuous watch on vital signs and the bispectral index readings. It is essential that from the initiation of intubation and IV drip infusion to extubation and then finally transfer from the ICU to the step-down unit that the anesthesiologist remain at the helm of the patient's care.

A patient profile is maintained with demographic and clinical information reflective of the burn injury and related opioid analgesia interventions. Specific data include the patient's age, type and degree of burn injury, burn size and location, injury severity score, duration of narcotic use prior to detoxification intervention and detailed daily narcotic consumption measured in morphine equivalent units, both prior to and after URODA, and length of hospital stay (**Box 1**).

Box 1	
Example of demographic data collected for patients undergoing URODA procedure	
Average age	31 years old
Average length of stay for URODA process	1 to 2 days
Average total burn surface area	38%
Average injury severity score	30
Average days of opioid use prior to URODA	672 days
Average opioid use PRIOR to URODA	>200 morphine equivalent units daily
Average opioid use AFTER URODA	<25 morphine equivalent units

The successful outcome for the authors' patients is multifold: the substantial decrease in opioid demand for pain control to less than one-eighth of the required morphine equivalent units (MEUs) prior to URODA, perceived improvement of self-esteem, and lightening of mood and affect as demonstrated by patient comments such as, "I can begin living again," "Food tastes so different when you can feed yourself," and "What really made me want to change was when my son asked me if I was going to have to take pills the rest of my life. . .and now I am living without pain medication!"

In reviewing experiences with the URODA protocol process, some valuable lessons were learned. It is imperative that health care providers take full responsibility for establishing the protocol and tailoring it to the needs of their target patient population, conduct a comprehensive history and physical examination, and maintain vigilance over all prescriptions and interventions. These requirements were evident when nurses not familiar with the URODA protocol and process contacted available or in-house resident physicians not associated with the protocol rather than the primary attending physicians such as the anesthesiologist. Nursing staff needed to be ICU-trained and experienced and possess critical thinking skills with the ability to identify and respond to at-risk conditions such as heart block and cardiac arrest as well as symptoms of pulmonary hypertension. Furthermore, caution should be exercised when administering cardiorespiratory medications and sedatives postextubation because of the heightened sensitivity to the same opioid doses the patient was taking prior to undergoing the URODA procedure.

Other difficulties were encountered. Some necessary monitoring equipment was not always available and challenges with hospital/regional medication shortages often required revision of the medication strategies. An example was when the facility phased out a specific awareness monitor used to assess depth of sedation and guide infusion rates. Coordination was required to compensate for the fact that the hospital no longer stocked these bispectral index supplies. Additionally, during the URODA study, a national shortage of propofol was encountered; therefore, increased dosing of ketamine and dexmedetomidine had to be used.

The goal in treating chronic burn-related pain is for the burn patient to reclaim control of his or her life and to be relieved of pain. There have been no complications with this protocol, and all patients have been more than satisfied with the results.[4] A multidisciplinary approach can be used in a burn center in conjunction with URODA to safely and effectively decrease opioid demands for the recovering burn patient.

Survival is not just living, but living a quality life. Patients must be treated like a loving member of your family. You would not want to see them in pain. The patient survived the burn injury, the dressing changes, the wound care, the surgeries, and the protracted rehabilitation course. There is now opportunity to optimize their pain management plan, maximizing pain control while minimizing opioid dependence and the debilitating withdrawal symptoms as much as possible.

REFERENCES

1. Argoff CE, Turk DC, Benzon HT, et al. Major opioids and chronic opioid therapy. Philadelphia: Mosby Elsevier; 2008.
2. Opioid related disorders. In: Moore DP, Jefferson JW, editors. Handbook of medical psychiatry. 2nd edition. St. Louis (MO): Mosby, Inc; 2004.
3. Wax PM, Ruha AM. Withdrawal syndromes. Opioid withdrawal. In: Irwin RS, Rippe JM, editors. Irwin and Rippe's intensive care medicine. Philadelphia (PA): Lippincott Williams & Wilkins; 2003.
4. Maani CV, DeSocio PA, Jansen RK, et al. Use of ultra rapid opioid detoxification in the treatment of us military burn casualties. J Trauma 2011;71:S114–9.
5. Stotts AL, Dodrill CL, Kosten TR. Opioid dependence treatment: options in pharmacotherapy. Expert Opin Pharmacother 2009;10:1727–40.
6. O'Connor PG, Kosten TR. Rapid and ultrarapid opioid detoxification techniques. JAMA 1998;279(3):229–34.

Battlefield Pain Control: Forging Ahead by Building on the Past

Christopher V. Maani, MD, MC, US Army

KEYWORDS

- Pain management • Combat casualties
- Battlefield medicine • Analgesics

Regardless of how we opine on the current state of health care reform, most would agree that pain management is a right, not a privilege. Both the civilian patients we care for every day and the wounded warriors in our military deserve our very best efforts when it comes to controlling their pain and relieving their suffering. Solving the problem of excessive pain may prove more challenging in military populations than in civilian populations. Both physical and emotional suffering are problematic in survivors of combat-related injuries caused by explosions. Patients who experience combat-related blasts have more extensive physical injuries and greater pain severity than soldiers and civilians without blast injuries. **Fig. 1** is an exemplar of the extent of injuries commonly seen in blast patients. Additionally, those with combat-related burn injuries require larger opioid doses for pain than soldiers and civilians with nonblast injuries. Although the severity of injuries requires the implementation of sophisticated and intensive pain management strategies that are often cited as major health care expenditures, pain management is about much more than just dollars and cents.

Reduction of unnecessary pain and suffering is a cornerstone of medicine. Inadequate pain management is something we must act upon. The burden of pain is enough to encumber or overwhelm an individual when not treated well. Along with the coincident and inherent mental anguish of being in pain at any given moment, there are long-term sequelae as well. These may include posttraumatic stress disorder, depression, nonrestorative sleep patterns, and of course, chronic pain syndromes. Even the ability to perform activities of daily living can be compromised when pain cannot be managed appropriately. Pain management can be a potential problem for thousands of new patients each year.

The opinions or assertions contained herein are the private views of the authors and are not to be construed as official or as reflecting the views of the Department of the Army or the Department of Defense.

Department of Anesthesiology, United States Army Institute of Surgical Research and Army Burn Center, Brooke Army Medical Center, 3400 Rawley East Chambers Avenue, Fort Sam Houston, TX 78234, USA

E-mail address: Christopher.Maani@us.army.mil

Perioperative Nursing Clinics 7 (2012) 83–88
doi:10.1016/j.cpen.2011.12.001
1556-7931/12/$ – see front matter Published by Elsevier Inc.

periopnursing.theclinics.com

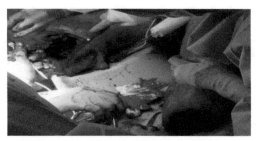

Fig. 1. Bilateral below-knee amputations in a far-forward setting following explosive blast injury.

Thousands of war fighters have suffered severe burn wounds and/or other trauma injuries secondary to the increased use of explosive weapons by enemy insurgents in Iraq and Afghanistan. Over 80% of American casualties are transported from Baghdad to Germany with uncontrolled pain.[1] Severe to excruciating pain often continues during the hospitalizations of these noble men and women injured in combat-related duty while serving their country. US war fighters with severe combat injuries such as significant burns, broken bones, penetrating soft-tissue injuries, and amputations must undergo frequent wound care sessions as part of their recovery. Whether it is the time-honored unit dose of morphine, 10 mg, or the state-of-the-art technology of immersive virtual therapy, successful analgesia reduces pain and suffering while improving outcomes and the patient's quality of life.

Conventional pain management techniques often are staid and need both improvement and enhancement. It is easy to see why, considering the most common prehospital pain medication: intramuscular (IM) or intravenous (IV) morphine. IM administration does not lend itself to easy titration, whereas IV titration is more feasible. However, both routes of administration require needles and requisite disposal of sharps. These routes also imply a need for exposure of the casualty; a problem in hypothermic trauma victims or soldiers in a tactical and potentially chemical environment. Morphine-induced respiratory and cardiovascular depression can also be especially challenging in this patient cohort that is prone to shock and hemorrhage.

Despite the many challenges in pain management, modern-day practices and possibilities are getting better. For example, available improvements beyond IM/IV morphine include oral administration of nonsteroidal anti inflammatory medications and acetaminophen/paracetamol. These can be bundled into a "combat pill pack," which incidentally may also include broad-spectrum antibiotics such as levofloxacin in an effort to stem infectious risks. Other currently available pain medications include the fentanyl lollipop, the opioid hydromorphone, and racemic ketamine. Although ketamine has historically been used primarily in the settings of emergency departments, pediatrics, and burns, the widespread battlefield and military use of ketamine in recent conflicts may result in mainstreaming its use again.[2,3]

There are also pharmaceutical products in the developmental pipeline that have yet to receive US Food and Drug Administration (FDA) clearance. Transdermal patient-controlled analgesia uses iontophoretic principles to maximize drug delivery. Recent technological advancements involving nanotechnology and the "pain vaccine" carry the potential to provide prolonged benefit, with analgesic durations lasting from hours to days at a time without the negative sequelae of opioids. Perhaps the most promising potential medication is S-ketamine—lauded by many as the next silver bullet in pain control. Although this claim may be too optimistic, an intentional and thorough approach is warranted to fully investigate its utility for battlefield application. The S-stereoisomer of ketamine seems to be more potent than the racemate, and it has fewer of the negative side effects often attributed to the R-isomer and the currently FDA-approved form of RS-ketamine. Given the current human use of S-ketamine over the last 2 decades in countries such as Germany, Brazil, India, and the Netherlands, its introduction into the United States, Britain, and Canada seems likely and is eagerly anticipated by many clinicians, military and civilian alike.

Current pain control considerations even include topical applications such as lidocaine patches for rib fractures. There is not much in the way of rigorously collected scientific data, but there have been several anecdotal accounts of success with this attractive analgesic option for prehospital or combat pain. Transcutaneous electrical nerve stimulation units and surface ultrasound have also been considered for their analgesic potential. These technologies could benefit patients with injuries ranging from isolated extremity injury to musculoskeletal pain of the torso, and there is a possibility that these are viable alternatives to the staple narcotic regimen still often encountered today. Battlefield acupuncture is yet another alternative. Popularized by US Air Force physician Dr Richard Niemtzow circa 2002, this simple technique requires only minimal training and very small, portable gold needles that barely penetrate the skin and do not require standard sharps disposal (**Fig. 2**). Other advantages include decreased incidence of adverse effects or contraindications and limiting exposure of the casualty. Whereas battlefield acupuncture has been reported to afford analgesia lasting up to 3 days, even several hours of pain relief are welcome.

"The Cadillac of pain control" is a phrase often used to describe regional anesthesia techniques. Although many peripheral nerve blocks (PNBs) may not be practical for first-responder care or self-aid, they do provide an excellent alternative to conventional multimodal therapy. Often requiring relatively minimal supplies (local anesthetic solution with stimulating needle, nerve stimulator, prep solution and sterile gloves), single-shot nerve blocks can afford patients analgesic benefits in excess of 18 to 24 hours. The simplicity and small logistical footprint of the PNB is demonstrated in **Fig. 3**. The main advantages include decreased opioid consumption, decreased nausea and vomiting, and increased patient awareness and satisfaction as

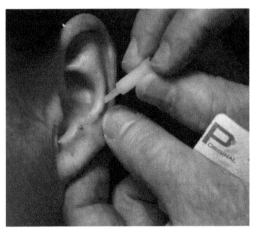

Fig. 2. Acupuncture or Auricular Semi-Permanent gold needles being placed in the ear for battlefield acupuncture.

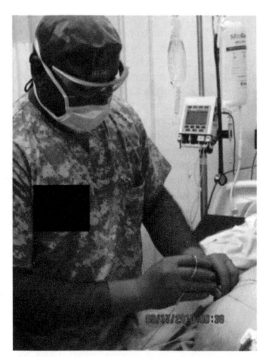

Fig. 3. Regional anesthesia on a combat-wounded soldier in a far-forward setting.

exemplified by the patient in **Fig. 4**. Within military and strategic/tactical consider-ations, PNBs offer an alternative that can mean the difference between injured soldiers ambulating themselves or having to be carried off by two or more fellow soldiers (further decreasing mission effective force or fighting strength).

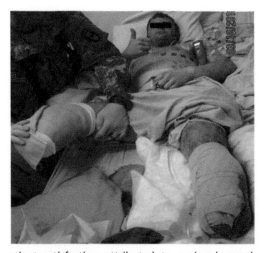

Fig. 4. Improved patient satisfaction attributed to regional anesthesia on a combat-wounded soldier in a far-forward setting.

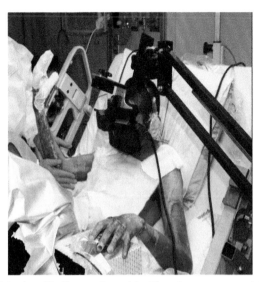

Fig. 5. Immersive virtual reality therapy to assist with pain management during burn wound care.

Seemingly a page out of a futuristic science fiction movie, immersive virtual reality (iVR) therapy is finding its way into the mainstream management of even the most complicated and severe pain. Long held in regard as the worst pain possible, burn pain seems to respond well to this new technology (**Fig. 5**). Because it harnesses technology and "virtual analgesia" science in lieu of more standard sedative pharmacotherapeutics, iVR analgesia does not cloud the patient's thinking, judgment, or consciousness like narcotic analgesics. This property becomes even more critical when air evacuation is involved, because patients are often undermedicated in an effort to stave off cardiorespiratory problems. Additional research is needed to confirm the efficacy and expand the availability of iVR, not only in the burn and trauma units, but also as far forward on the modern battlefield as possible, for example during medical evacuations and eventually even farther forward to combat support hospitals (CSHs) and forward surgical teams (FSTs). In its ultimate evolution, iVR could be as portable as a pair of glasses with head-mounted display capability and wireless technology. Although not usable under fire and during active firefights, iVR could be used to provide analgesia during evacuation to an FST or a CSH. iVR could also be useful during painful procedures during a soldier's stay at the FST or CSH facilities and during the evacuation to level 4 and level 5 facilities. By satisfying the military's request for battlefield interventions that minimally cloud the decision-making process, new therapeutic modalities such as iVR analgesia have the potential to impact on functional unit capability and mission accomplishment by minimizing sedation, maximizing pain control, and helping the combat-injured return to duty sooner.

More research and development are needed to study and validate these possibilities. Pain research will continue to light the way forward for pain clinicians and their patients alike. The interplay of suboptimal pain management and its effects on day-to-day activities cannot be underestimated. Society pays the bill for pain in the currency of work hours lost, health care dollars spent, and lives disrupted. Many times these lives are completely uprooted and entire families are destroyed. The problems these patients and their loved ones face on a daily basis are a reminder of this moral imperative: the need for us to continue our efforts to improve pain management and to provide our patients an escape from the dire consequences of poor pain control.

REFERENCES

1. Buckenmaier CC 3rd, Rupprecht C, McKnight G, et al. Pain following battlefield injury and evacuation: a survey of 110 casualties from the wars in Iraq and Afghanistan. Pain Med 2009;10(8):1487–96.
2. Guldner GT, Petinaux B, Clemens P, et al. Ketamine for procedural sedation and analgesia by nonanesthesiologists in the field: a review for military health care providers. Mil Med 2006;171(6):484–90.
3. Mercer SJ. 'The Drug of War'–a historical review of the use of Ketamine in military conflicts. J R Nav Med Serv 2009;95(3):145–50.

Pressure Ulcers in the Burned Patient: Perioperative Considerations

Sarah K. Shingleton, MS, RN, CCRN, CCNS

KEYWORDS

- Burn • Decubitus • Perioperative • Pressure sore
- Pressure ulcer • Pressure ulcer prevention

Pressure ulcers are a serious complication across healthcare settings and are associated with pain, disability, decreased quality of life, prolonged length of stay, and increased costs.[1–3] A pressure ulcer is a localized injury as a result of unrelieved pressure, often in combination with friction or shear, to the skin or underlying tissue.[4,5] A pressure ulcer generally occurs over a bony prominence, but may be associated with medical devices such as oxygen tubing, nasogastric tubes, and positioning devices.[2,6,7]

Burned individuals are a unique subset of patients at risk for pressure ulcer development; however, the scope of the pressure ulcer problem in burned patients has not been well-defined in the literature and current burn care practices must largely rely on established guidelines for pressure ulcer risk assessment, prevention, and treatment for nonburned individuals.[2] A unit-specific analysis of pressure ulcer prevalence from 2007 to 2009 described a facility-acquired prevalence in burn patients to be 6.2% in 2007, 9.9% in 2008, and 6.0% in 2009.[7] However, the results may not be truly representative because burn patients comprised a small subset.[7]

Focus on pressure ulcer prevalence and prevention has been increased over the last decade and has attracted the attention of many national patient safety and quality organizations such as The Joint Commission, the Institute for Healthcare Improvement, and the US Agency for Healthcare Research and Quality.[7,8] A 2006 review of the literature estimated that approximately 60,000 patients per year die as a result of complications related to pressure ulcers and that the associated cost to treat these wounds is approximately \$11 billion.[5,9] As of October 1, 2008, the Centers for

Disclaimer: The opinions or assertions contained herein are the private views of the author and are not to be construed as official or as reflecting the views of the Department of the Army or the Department of Defense.

US Army Institute of Surgical Research, 3698 Chambers Pass, Fort Sam Houston, TX 78234-6315, USA

E-mail address: sarah.k.shingleton@amedd.army.mil

Medicare and Medicaid Services no longer reimburse healthcare facilities for the related costs of healthcare-associated pressure ulcers.[7,10]

It is essential that healthcare professionals be aware of the risks and implications of pressure ulcer development in the patient populations served in their settings. Pressure ulcer development may begin any time a patient experiences skin or tissue compromise, resulting in skin breakdown. A review of the literature shows that pressure ulcers are commonly discussed with regard to long-term, rehabilitation, and acute care settings.[5] However, limited literature is available with regard to the perioperative and burn patient populations.[2,5] This article discusses the primary causes of and risk factors associated with pressure ulcer development, unique considerations when providing care for burned individuals, perioperative risk factors for pressure ulcer development, and methods for pressure redistribution and prevention of ulcers that could develop during operative procedures.

PRESSURE ULCER FORMATION AND RISK FACTORS

Patients are assumed to be at greatest risk for pressure ulcer development during the intraoperative period.[11] Operative procedures place even the healthiest individuals at risk for pressure ulcer development; thus, the risk is exacerbated in surgical patients experiencing other acute or chronic illnesses. Operation-related tissue damage and pressure ulcer formation may not be clearly evident in the postoperative patient for up to 3 days postprocedure when the ulcer is staged.[5,12] The most common presentation of an intraoperatively associated pressure ulcer is that of a suspected deep tissue injury, which presents as a purple or maroon localized area of intact skin or a blood-filled blister, although breakdown may present later as a different stage[4,5,13,14] (**Table 1**). These lesions generally develop on the muscle of a bony prominence and are a result of underlying tissue damage.[13] Common bony prominences particularly at risk include the ankles, coccyx, elbows, greater trochanters, heels, ischial tuberosities, knees, occiput, sacrum, scapulae, shoulders, and areas of the spine.

Pressure ulcers are caused by a compression of soft tissue between a bony prominence and another surface such as a bed, operating room table, or device. The consequential damage is a result of compromised blood flow to the skin and soft tissues. Tissue tolerance is described as the ability of the skin and underlying structures to tolerate the effects of pressure without adverse effects, such as skin and tissue injury.[5,15] Tissue tolerance is a major factor in pressure ulcer development and varies greatly as a result of an individual patient's skin condition and risk factors. Factors affecting an individual patient's risk for pressure ulcer development are generally categorized into 2 major groups: extrinsic and intrinsic factors.

Extrinsic risk factors for pressure ulcer development include pressure, friction, shear, and moisture. When external pressure exceeds the normal capillary filling pressure of approximately 32 mmHg, local blood flow is occluded and the result is tissue ischemia. Muscle has been shown to be more sensitive to pressure than skin, and damage may take place before ulceration appears on the skin. Shear is a force that results in a sliding motion between the planes of an object, for example, when skin is pulled in 1 direction and bone in another while turning a patient. This motion may also cause constriction of blood flow to the area, placing the patient at risk for pressure ulcer development. Friction is a mechanical force directed against the skin's epidermis. This can happen when the head or heels are allowed to drag across a sheet during repositioning or on the sacrum as the head of bed is elevated. Moisture is another factor placing the skin at risk for breakdown. When skin is excessively moist as a result of urinary incontinence or excessive wound drainage, for example, tissue tensile strength is decreased and maceration can easily occur. Each of these

Table 1	
Pressure ulcer stage description	
Stage I	• Intact skin with non-blanchable redness of a localized area (usually a bony prominence).
	• In darker skinned patients, often the area does not blanch; look for a color difference from the surrounding skin.
	• Area may be painful, firm, soft, warmer or cooler compared to adjacent tissue.
Stage II	• Partial thickness loss of dermis appearing as a shallow, open ulcer with a red or pink wound bed without slough.
	• May also present as an intact or open/ruptured serum-filled blister.
Stage III	• Full thickness tissue loss; subcutaneous fat may be visable but bone, tendon or muscle are not exposed.
	• May also include undermining and/or tunneling.
Stage IV	• Full thickness tissue loss accompanied by exposed bone, tendon or muscle. Slough or eschar may cover portions of the wound bed.
	• Often have undermining and tunneling.
Unstageable	• Full thickness tissue loss in which the base of the wound is covered by slough (yellow, tan, gray, green or brown) and/or eschar (tan, brown or black).
	• Until enough slough or eschar can be removed to expose the wound base, the true depth and stage cannot be determined.
Suspected Deep Tissue Injury	• Localized area of discolored skin, often appearing maroon or purple, or blood-filled blister as a result of shear/pressure injury to the underlying soft tissue or muscle. The discolored area may be preceded by tissue that feels painful, warmer, cooler, firm, boggy, or mushy compared to adjacent tissue.
	• Similar to Stage I ulcers, sDTI may be difficult to detect in patients with dark skin tones.
	• sDTI may further evolve and become covered by thin eschar and evolution of the wound may be rapid.

Data from Pressure ulcer stages revised by the National Pressure Ulcer Advisory Panel. Ostomy Wound Manage 2007; 53(3):30–1.

factors is not only of particular concern in older adults, but also in burned patients due, in part, to large insensible fluid losses and the necessary use of positioning devices that have potential to rub against the skin.

Intrinsic risk factors affect the capability of the skin and supporting structures to respond to pressure, friction, and shear forces. These include advanced age, impaired mobility, sensory deficits, nutritional deficiencies, hemodynamic alterations, and comorbid conditions. Burned patients often have many of the following factors identified as affecting tissue perfusion: Medications (eg, steroids and vasoactive medications), comorbidities (eg, peripheral vascular disease and diabetes mellitus), impaired regulation in body temperature, edema formation, decreased hemoglobin and hematocrit levels, obesity, low serum protein, alcohol and nicotine abuse, and decreased blood pressure.[2,5,16,17]

RISK IN THE BURN-INJURED PATIENT

Burn patients have many risk factors that have been shown through literature and clinical practice to be risk factors for pressure ulcer development (**Fig. 1**). After the initial burn injury, patients quickly experience massive fluid shifts as plasma volume is

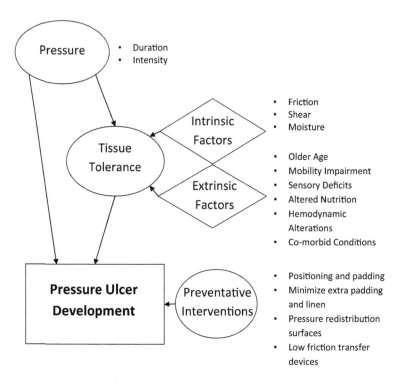

Fig. 1. Factors influencing pressure ulcer development in the surgical burn patient.

lost and fluid collects in the burned tissue. Patients with greater than a 20% total body surface area (TBSA) burn require formal fluid resuscitation in order to prevent hypovolemic shock, also known as "burn shock," and to maintain blood flow and oxygenation to the vital organs. In addition, burn patients often experience decreased mobility during the initial management phase. Numerous procedures, including intubation, central venous and arterial catheter placement, and initial wound care, are performed during initial management which require analgesia, sedation, and frequently, paralytics. Immobility, hypovolemia, and decreased oxygenation to the tissue have all been shown to be major risk factors for pressure ulcer development.

Burn patients develop generalized edema during fluid resuscitation that usually peaks 2 to 3 days post burn. Edema is thought to be a risk factor for pressure ulcer formation in that it puts more distance between the capillary bed and the cells, thereby reducing the rate of diffusion of oxygen and nutrients to the skin and supporting tissues.[16,18] Patients must be continually evaluated for skin breakdown during this time, particularly with regard to devices such as positioning splints and endotracheal tube holders, because increasing edema may cause a device to become too tight. Burn patients also experience large insensible fluid losses through open wounds, thus contributing to increased moisture to uninjured skin and placing it at risk for maceration and skin breakdown as well. In addition, some types of wound dressings are required to be moistened with sterile water or antimicrobial solutions several times per day to prevent wound desiccation, again, placing uninjured skin at risk for breakdown.

Inadequate nutrition is known to be a significant risk factor for pressure ulcer development across settings. However, limited evidence has shown that the use of vitamin and mineral supplementation, in the absence of real deficiency, is helpful in the prevention and treatment of pressure ulcers.[9,17] Burn patients are unique in that they are at great risk of micronutrient deficiencies and experience an extended hypermetabolic state, placing them at a significant risk for inadequate nutrition and protein malnutrition. Resting energy expenditure in the burned patient may be double that of normal as a result of hypermetabolism and the delivery of adequate calories, protein, amino acids, and micronutrients is critical to wound healing.[2,19] Enteral hyperalimentation is preferred and ideally begun early via either nasogastric or nasojejunal feeding tubes. At a minimum, all burn patients should receive a daily vitamin and mineral supplementation.[2] When possible, interruptions in enteral feedings are minimized and patients often are fed until just before surgery and, in some burn centers, may receive postpyloric feedings throughout the case.

Burn patients are at a great risk for developing burn wound infection, sepsis, and multiple organ dysfunction syndrome.[2,19] The major cause of death in burn patients with greater than 20% TBSA burns who survive after the first 24 hours is multiple organ dysfunction syndrome.[19] Patients may require additional fluid resuscitation and the use of multiple vasopressors to manage their septic shock. The use of vasopressors in an already low flow state further decreases perfusion to the skin and tissues, thereby placing the patient at an increased risk for pressure ulcer formation.

Data from the National Burn Repository from 1999 to 2008 revealed that adults over the age of 60 comprised approximately 12% of all patients treated at participating burn centers.[20] Although this is a fairly small percentage of patients, older adults who are burned have higher complication and mortality rates compared with other age groups and have been found to have the highest incidence of pressure ulcer development in the general adult population.[5,20] The older adult is at high risk of sustaining tissue injury intraoperatively because of age-related skin changes, which include a thinner dermis, decreased elasticity, and decreased collagen, muscle, and adipose tissue. These characteristics make older patients not just susceptible to pressure ulcers, but also to increased bruising, skin tears, and delayed healing.[5]

Early excision and skin grafting is the standard of care for patients will full-thickness burn injuries. Burn patients with large TBSA injuries require multiple operative procedures for excision of the burn and placement of skin grafts or another temporary wound covering. Skin grafts are most commonly obtained from the patient and are termed "autografts." Often, temporary wound coverings are used when adequate donor skin is not available, as in the case of large TBSA burns. During the procedures, burn patients are under anesthesia, immobilized for extended periods of time, and experience large amounts of fluid and blood loss resulting in decreased tissue perfusion. Postoperatively, bulky dressings and splints are placed with the goal of protecting the skin grafts and need to be placed with enough pressure to aid in hemostasis in the grafted wounds and donor sites. However, edema formation is a common issue postoperatively and if dressings are placed too tightly, increased pressure on the skin and underlying structures may occur. Postoperative dressings and splints generally remain in place for 3 to 5 days, depending on several factors, including surgeon preference.

INTRAOPERATIVE CONSIDERATIONS

Positioning is a key component of surgical care. The body must be adequately positioned on the OR bed and care must be taken to maintain proper body alignment to minimize the risk of potential complications and skin injuries. Improper positioning may result in complications with blood pressure and venous return, resulting in inadequate tissue perfusion.[5] The position chosen for a surgical procedure depends on the type of procedure to be performed, the need for exposure of the surgical site, the surgeon's preference, the anesthesia provider's needs, and the individual patient's needs.[5,13] The most frequent positions used during burn surgery are supine, prone, and lateral.

Ideally, all burn injured patients should be repositioned during surgical procedures. O'Connell[21] found in 1 study of surgical patients that procedures lasting longer than 4 hours "triple the risk of tissue damage.". Burn surgeries may last up to 4 hours and potentially longer. Although large position changes may not always be reasonable during certain procedures, it is generally possible to frequently reposition areas such as the head, feet, and arms. Multiple positions are frequently used during any 1 burn surgery, depending on the patient's condition. For example, excision and grafting may be required on both the anterior and posterior aspects of the body. Also, the posterior trunk is a frequent choice for donor skin to be harvested, often requiring the patient to first be placed in the prone position and then repositioned supine.

Anesthesia places the patient at risk for multiple complications as common agents used may result in depression of the autonomic nervous system and vasodilatation. Vasodilatation is reflected by a decrease in blood pressure which in turn leads to a decrease in tissue perfusion. It is felt that intraoperative hypotension, reflected by a diastolic blood pressure less than 60 mmHg, places patients at risk for pressure ulcer development postoperatively.[11,12]

A consideration that has not been well defined in the literature but is a possible risk factor for skin breakdown is the use of skin preparation solutions during surgery. Although this is a critical step in the preparation of a patient for skin incision and the prevention of surgical site infection, it is possible that pooling of prep solution under the patient during surgery, in combination with wound exudate and other fluid losses, could result in skin maceration. Combined with friction and shear forces during repositioning, for example, skin is at risk for breakdown.[12]

SKIN ASSESSMENT AND RISK DETERMINATION

Pressure ulcer risk assessment is an important intervention that identifies patients at risk for breakdown and aids the interdisciplinary team in developing a plan of care aimed at prevention. The Braden Scale for Predicting Pressure Sore Risk is a validated tool available for clinicians and is widely used across healthcare settings to identify risk and guide preventative interventions.[22] The scale consists of 6 subscales including sensory perception, moisture, activity, mobility, nutrition, and friction and shear. Possible scores range from 6 to 23 with lower scores suggesting higher risk (**Table 2**). Although use of the Braden Scale is not intended for determining intraoperative pressure ulcer risk, it can aid the perioperative nurse in determining whether the patient has a baseline risk for pressure ulcer development.[11,12]

Table 2	
Braden scale risk levels	
Risk level	Value
At risk	15–18
Moderate risk	13–14
High risk	10–12
Very high risk	≤9

Data from Bergstrom N, Braden B, Kemp M, et al. Predicting pressure ulcer risk: a multisite study of the predictive validity of the Braden Scale. Nurs Res 1998;47:261–9.

Thorough skin assessment of the burn patient should be completed by the perioperative nurse. On the day of surgery, burn patients often do not have their dressings changed before the procedure; therefore, the assessment may need to be completed by the OR nurse when dressings are removed before preparation of the skin. A visual inspection of potential pressure points should be completed both before and after the procedure. The nurse should note any skin breakdown or discoloration at pressure points and also look for any skin complications such as rash, maceration, infection, and venous insufficiency.[5] Any significant findings should be included in the handoff communication process each time there is a transfer in care, such as from the surgical suite to the postanesthesia care unit.[12]

CONSIDERATIONS FOR PREVENTION AND RECOMMENDATIONS

Guidelines from the American Association of PeriOperative Registered Nurses (AORN), "Recommended practices for positioning the patient in the perioperative setting," suggest that patients should be repositioned every 2 hours to prevent continuous pressure on pressure points and decrease the risk of adverse physiologic responses.[5,13] When repositioning patients in the OR, a lateral transfer device that minimizes friction and shear should be used to ensure safety for the staff and patient. Pressure-reliving positioning devices are available in different shapes and sizes and should be used instead of rolled sheets and towels.[13]

Pressure redistribution surfaces are widely used in the operative environment as a replacement for a standard OR table mattress. These devices are not designed to relieve or reduce pressure, but to redistribute pressure by reducing the interface tissue pressure. The chosen overlay should allow for the patient to be immersed in the surface, but also needs be firm enough to prevent bottoming out which occurs when the device is no longer preventing direct pressure between the patient and the OR table or bed.[5,23] There are several types of support surfaces available ranging from foam and gel overlays to dynamic air overlays that are operated by a mechanical pump.[5]

Gel overlays can be placed directly over the standard OR mattress and are made of a viscoelastic polymer type material. This type of overlay helps to minimize friction, shear, and bottoming out and should be used with the polymer side in contact with the patient. Overlays that combine the pressure redistribution properties of polymer gel with an electrosurgical grounding pad are available and help to distribute heat evenly, preventing hot areas on the pad. However, it is challenging to keep these combination gel pads dry when using them during burn surgery owing to large fluid and blood losses. Static air overlays are another type of pad that allows for air movement through multiple chambers as the patient lies on the overlay. This type of overlay must be reinflated periodically to maintain pressure redistribution.

Dynamic air overlays are commonly used outside of the OR and include low-air-loss beds, air-fluidized mattresses, and alternating pressure mattresses. They require a mechanical pump to produce alternating inflation and deflation. Although dynamic overlays may provide better pressure redistribution than gel overlays and standard OR mattresses, they are not commonly used in intraoperatively because of potential electrical problems, asepsis, and the possibility of body movement.[13]

Consideration should be given to minimizing the use of extra pads, blankets, and warming blankets in conjunction with pressure redistribution surfaces. A common misconception is that extra layers of linen add to patient comfort and minimize moisture when, in fact, they may contribute to increased skin moisture and interfere with the surface's ability to conform around the patient. Layers either beneath the overlay or between the patient and overlay should be minimized or avoided because they decrease the effectiveness of the overlay and may cause increased pressure.[5] The use of too many blankets or pads on top of or beneath the patient may cause the capillary pressure to rise over 32 mmHg, thus increasing the risk for poor tissue perfusion intraoperatively.[13]

SUMMARY

All surgical patients should be considered at risk for developing pressure ulcers because of the multiple factors often encountered intraoperatively including the length of surgery, hemodynamic status as affected by anesthesia, immobility, and sensory deficits. Burn patients are especially at risk for further skin and tissue injury as a result of the many risk factors they have preoperatively from their injuries. Key components of a perioperative pressure injury prevention strategy include thorough skin assessments, interventions to reduce shear and friction during patient positioning and transfer, and use of pressure redistribution surfaces and overlays. A collaborative approach involving the multidisciplinary burn team is vital in the ongoing care of the burned patient and is essential to the achievement of positive outcomes and maintenance of a safe patient environment.

REFERENCES

1. Allman RM, Goode PS, Burst N, et al. Pressure ulcers, hospital complications, and disease severity: impact on hospital costs and length of stay. Adv Wound Care 1999;12:22–30.
2. Gordon MD, Gottschlich MM, Helvig EI, et al. Review of evidenced-based practice for the prevention of pressure sores in burn patients. J Burn Care Rehabil 2004;25:388–410.
3. Reddy M, Keast D, Fowler E, et al. Pain in pressure ulcers. Ostomy Wound Manage 2003;49(4 Suppl):30–5.
4. Pressure ulcer stages revised by the National Pressure Ulcer Advisory Panel. Ostomy Wound Manage 2007;53(3):30–1.
5. Walton-Geer PS. Prevention of pressure ulcers in the surgical patient. AORN J 2009;89:538–52.
6. Black JM, Cuddigan JE, Walko MA, et al. Medical device related pressure ulcers in hospitalized patients. Int Wound J 2010;7:358–65.
7. VanGilder C, Amlung S, Harrison P, et al. Results of the 2008-2009 International Pressure Ulcer Prevalence Survey and a 3-year, acute care, unit-specific analysis. Ostomy Wound Manage 2009;55(11):39–45.
8. Lyder CH, Ayello EA. Pressure ulcers: a patient safety issue. In: Hughes RG, editor. Patient safety and quality: an evidence-based handbook for nurses. Rockville (MD): Agency for Healthcare Research and Quality (US); 2008.

9. Reddy M, Gill SS, Rochon PA. Preventing pressure ulcers: a systematic review. JAMA 2006;296:974–84.

10. Hospital-acquired conditions (present on admission indicator). The Centers for Medicare and Medicaid Services. Available at: http://www.cms.gov/HospitalAcqCond/. Accessed May 29, 2011.

11. Bergstrom N. The Braden Scale for Predicting Pressure Sore Risk: reflections on the perioperative period. J Wound Ostomy Continence Nurs 2005;32(2):79–80.

12. Price MC, Whitney JD, King CA, et al. Development of a risk assessment tool for intraoperative pressure ulcers. J Wound Ostomy Continence Nurs 2005;32:19–30.

13. Recommended practices for positioning the patient in the perioperative setting. Perioperative Standards and Recommended Practices. Denver: AORN, INC; 2008. p. 497–520.

14. Position statement: pressure ulcer staging. Wound Ostomy and Continence Nurses Society. Available at: http://www.wocn.org/pdfs/WOCN_Library/Position_Statements/PressureUlcerStaging.pdf. Accessed May 29, 2011.

15. Pieper B. Mechanical forces: pressure, shear, and friction. In: Bryant R, Nix D, editors. Acute & chronic wounds: current management concepts. 3rd edition. St Louis: Mosby; 2007. p. 205–34.

16. McCord S, McElvain V, Sachdeva R, et al. Risk factors associated with pressure ulcers in the pediatric intensive care unit. J Wound Ostomy Continence Nurs 2004; 31(4):179–83.

17. Lyder CH. Pressure ulcer prevention and management. JAMA 2003;289:223–6.

18. Schue RM, Langemo DK. Pressure ulcer prevalence and incidence and a modification of the Braden Scale for a rehabilitation unit. J Wound Ostomy Continence Nurs 1998;25(1):36–43.

19. Greenhalgh DG, Saffle JR, Holmes JHI, et al. American Burn Association Consensus Conference to define sepsis and infection in burns. J Burn Care Res 2007; 28:776–90.

20. Miller SF, Jeng JC, Bessey P, et al. National burn repository 2009 report: dataset 5.0. 2009. Available at: http://www.ameriburn.org/2009NBRAnnualReport.pdf. Accessed May 29, 2011.

21. O'Connell MP. Positioning impact on the surgical patient. Nurs Clin North Am 2006;41(2):173–92.

22. Bergstrom N, Braden B, Kemp M, et al. Predicting pressure ulcer risk: a multisite study of the predictive validity of the Braden Scale. Nurs Res 1998;47:261–9.

23. Schultz A. Predicting and preventing pressure ulcers in surgical patients. AORN J 2005;81:986–1006.

A Burn Progressive Care Unit: Customized Care from Admission Through Discharge

Christina L. Moore, CPT, AN, BSN, Patricia M. Schmidt, CPT, AN, BSN, MHS*

KEYWORDS

• Nursing care • Burn unit • Progressive care • Burn recovery

Four East is a 24-bed burn progressive care unit (BPCU) located in the burn center of the Institute of Surgical Research, San Antonio Military Medical Center, Fort Sam Houston, Texas. Patients in the BPCU are transferred from the burn ICU (intensive care unit, BICU), admitted through the emergency department or the burn clinic, or are readmissions for surgical scar revisions. BPCU patients may arrive accompanied by the burn center's dedicated burn flight team, or SMART team (special medical augmentation response team), or with civilian personnel as transfers from other area hospitals. Criteria for direct admission to the BPCU are total body surface area (TBSA) burn of less than 20% with stable vital signs and lab values and minimal oxygen requirements.

ADMISSIONS

Patients who are directly admitted to the BPCU are evaluated in the emergency department or burn clinic prior to transfer. If patients arrive with the burn flight team they are admitted directly to the floor. After completion of admission paperwork and placing of an intravenous line, the patient is transferred to a shower cart so that nursing staff can easily move the patient from the bed into the shower room. Typically the patient receives oral narcotics for baseline pain control and is given intravenous narcotics throughout the shower, hydrotherapy, and debridement process as needed.

In the shower room, nursing staff use 4% chlorhexidine gluconate soap, sterile burn gauze pads, forceps, and scissors to remove any nonadherent tissue and blisters from the burn areas. Burn gauze pads are used like washcloths to scrub off any

The opinions or assertions contained herein are the private views of the authors and are not to be construed as official or as reflecting the views of the Department of the Army or the Department of Defense.
Burn Center 4 East, United States Army Institute of Surgical Research, 3698 Chambers Pass, Fort Sam Houston, TX 78234-6315, USA
* Corresponding author.
E-mail address: patricia.schmidt@amedd.army.mil

Perioperative Nursing Clinics 7 (2012) 99–105
doi:10.1016/j.cpen.2011.12.003
1556-7931/12/$ – see front matter Published by Elsevier Inc.

periopnursing.theclinics.com

additional loose tissue. Following this debridement the attending burn surgeon or surgical resident examines the patient's burns to determine the severity and location of the burns and initiates the wound care treatment and dressings that will best promote healing. Various dressings are used depending on the severity of the burn, size of the burn, and stage of wound healing. Daily dressing changes reduce the risk of developing infection and promote wound healing.

After initial wound care, patients and their families are oriented to their hospital room and the BPCU. Nurses work with the patient and family one-on-one, providing English and Spanish written handouts and verbal education about the burn wound's healing process and expectations for the hospital stay.

TRANSFERS

When BICU patients meet BPCU admission criteria, the multidisciplinary team identifies them as ready to transfer and orders are written initiating transfer to the BPCU. Patients and families often feel stress when transferring from the BICU; factors that cause this stress are personal or situational. Some personal factors may include knowledge, beliefs, values, goals, and commitments. The patient and family may be surprised by the initiation of the transfer if they have not been prepared, if staff have not communicated that the patient's condition is improving, or if staff have not emphasized the benefits of moving to the lower acuity of care. If the patient and family believe the patient still requires continuous monitoring, they may feel anxious about the move to a lower acuity of care because they believe their issues will not be addressed in a timely manner.

The BPCU staff assure the patient and family that the new unit has continuous monitoring capabilities for patients who require them and practices team nursing with hourly rounds, so at least one staff member has patient contact every hour of the day. Patients are also reassured that they will not be overlooked and that their goals for discharge are encouraged and supported.

Patient values can also have an effect on the transfer process; when a patient or family believes that transferring from one unit to another will change the quality of care, then there may be hesitancy or apprehension about the transfer. Also, if the patient believes his or her goals for progressing will not be met when transferred, unnecessary stress may be felt.

Patients and families may have developed relationships with the nursing staff from the BICU and feel a commitment from that staff. Transferring to another unit can lead to feelings of being abandoned by the BICU staff and apprehension about creating relationships with the BPCU staff. To help with the transition between BICU and BPCU, nursing staff from the BICU accompany the patient and family to introduce them to the new staff, and they visit often with the patient and family to see how they are doing after the transfer.

Situational factors stemming from the transfer event—change in physical environment and the support available—may also affect the stress level of the patient and family. Patients who view an ICU environment as safe, secure, and reassuring require adequate preparation prior to transfer to reduce their feelings of anxiety related to the transfer, whereas a patient who perceives the ICU as a stressful environment may view the transfer as welcoming.[1] Transfer from the BICU indicates that the patient's condition has improved, and the patient must be told this. The stress of immediate fear of dying may transition into stress related to living with long-term impairments.[1] Burn patients also experience this stress as they realize their long-term impairments, whether they were directly admitted to the BPCU or are being transferred from the BICU.

At the burn center, transfers are identified during morning multidisciplinary rounds. Input is received from the physician, physician's assistant, nursing staff, and rehabilitation representatives about the patient's readiness for transfer to the BPCU. Criteria for transfer include pain controlled without continuous narcotic or ketamine infusions, weaned from sedation and vasoactive medications, heart rate between 40 and 130 beats per minute, respiratory rate between 8 and 24 breaths per minute, oxygen saturation above 90% with supplemental oxygen, and systolic blood pressure higher than 90 mmHg. The BICU charge nurse notifies the BPCU charge nurse of the impending patient transfers after the BICU rounds, allowing the BPCU time to prepare for the transfer. The BPCU charge nurse assigns the patient to a nursing team of one registered nurse (RN) (the team leader), and one or two licensed vocational nurses (LVNs), notifies the RN team leader they will be receiving the transfer, and prepares a bed for the new patient. This early notification system allows the nursing team time to plan their schedule to manage the care of the patients already assigned to the team and transition the transferring patient and family with ease.

Transfers to the BPCU generally occur between noon and 3 PM; this window permits time for the patient to become familiar with the new environment and meet the BPCU staff before bedtime. Families of burn patients usually visit during daytime hours. Some accompany their loved one during transfer from the BICU, or they arrive to see the patient shortly thereafter. Visiting hours in the BPCU differ from those of the BICU; nursing staff explain to the patient and family that visiting hours are from 7 to 7:30 AM so that families may eat breakfast with the patient as well as assist the patient to eat, then the unit is closed to visitors from 7:30 AM to noon for multidisciplinary rounds and wound care. Visiting hours resume at noon and extend until 10 PM. Exceptions to the closed unit are made for preoperative visits and for family members to learn wound care prior to discharge. Having family members present during the transfer is comforting for the patient and affords the family opportunity to ask questions.[1]

As with direct admissions, nursing staff orient BICU transfer patients to the BPCU using the unit orientation care plan. The orientation includes introduction to the staff and team nursing system, as well as any information about unit policies including visiting hours, the practice of hourly rounds, the use of safety equipment like call bells, and nutrition support, which includes both the process of calling the kitchen to order meals and information about access to the refrigerator and snacks available to patients on the BPCU.

BPCU ROUTINE

In the BPCU, the goals of care are driven by the psychosocial and emotional needs of the patient: assist the patient with recovery, focus on wound healing, and prepare the patient and family for discharge. Patient education is a component of both psychosocial and emotional needs goals.[2]

Staffing on the BPCU varies depending on the patient census and the acuity of the patients on the unit. During a 12-hour shift, a team of one RN and one LVN may have from 3 to 6 patients and manage their patients' pain, provide monitoring, conduct wound care, and work closely with the physical and occupational therapists from the rehabilitation department to properly splint and elevate patients' limbs.

The BPCU conducts daily morning multidisciplinary rounds to include one or more physician, physician's assistant, clinical nurse specialist, case manager and/or social worker, nursing staff member, dietary representative, rehabilitation representative (physical therapist/occupational therapist), behavioral health representative, and chaplain. These rounds allow all personnel caring for the patient to present concerns, receive updates, and discuss the discharge plan for the patient. Daily rounds provide for all members of the care team to be active in the patient's plan of care and provide the patient and family with consistency in patient care.

A typical schedule includes the morning removal of the patient's dressings so that wound healing may be evaluated by multidisciplinary team members, followed by a daily shower and new dressings, then rehabilitation therapy, both in the room and in the rehabilitation gym. The patient's day usually begins before 6 AM and ends about 4 PM.

Throughout their hospital stay, burn patients begin to adapt to the challenges of recovery. Their healing skin and scars may cover joints, making daily activities that once were easy now challenging. Patients may need to relearn how to walk, brush their teeth, or hold utensils to eat, and they must also learn new skills like how to properly care for their healed skin after discharge.

NUTRITION

Burn patients are in a hypermetabolic state and require a continuous high-carbohydrate, high-protein diet. Patients who do not meet their daily requirements are frequently placed on tube feedings through a nasogastric or Dobbhoff tube. A majority of patients are placed on a calorie count plan until they meet or exceed their caloric intake for several days. Nursing staff encourage milk, supplement drinks, and food from home to help patients meet their nutritional goals. Water is not allowed because it reduces the patient's sodium levels and/or fills the patient's stomach, which results in not consuming enough food or supplements to meet caloric needs for the day. The patients who have an unrestricted diet are healed burn patients who have returned for various follow-up surgeries.[2]

SAME-DAY SURGERY

As burned skin matures, restrictive scars can form. Scarring is an individualized process with multiple factors influencing formation. Compliance with compression garments, splinting, and stretching devices for mouths or joints, and rehabilitative therapy are controllable factors; scar formation has a genetic component that is unknown until burned skin begins to heal. Keloids, hypertrophic scars, and contractures can form when the burned skin is replaced with excessive fibrosis formation and limiting skin compliance. To restore function to the burn patient, a scar contracture release or removal of the scar tissue is performed. Surgical releases and removal are commonly performed over areas of the body where a joint is affected such as fingers, elbows, shoulders, knees, neck, and chin.[3] Scar removal and releases reduce the continued production of tumor growth factors, and tension release from the procedure also reduces collagen production.

Reconstructive surgery patients come to the BPCU after admission through the same-day surgery department. The practice of keeping burn same-day surgery patients in the hospital differs from that for same-day surgery patients with other types of surgical procedures, who are discharged home within 24 hours postoperatively. Instead of sending patients home after surgery, they are kept on for 1 or 2 days to ensure their pain is appropriately managed and to be monitored for possible complications from the surgery.[4]

Because the scar revision procedures are performed on sensitive areas of the body like the nose, eyes, ears, neck, and hands, the patient and family, as well as licensed providers, are more comfortable having the patient monitored by experienced burn nursing staff during the postoperative phase. Nursing staff also assess the patient for dangerous swelling, difficulty voiding, and possible infection. They work with patients to control pain so that they are comfortable and pain is controlled with oral medications at the time of discharge. Same-day surgery patients go home with their surgical dressings in place with a scheduled burn clinic appointment for removal of the dressings.[4]

POSTOPERATIVE CARE

Patients received by direct admission through the burn clinic, emergency department, transfers from other facilities, burn flight team admission, or transfer from the BICU may require surgical intervention and postoperative care. Burn wounds and surgery are associated with significant pain. The nursing staff and providers work with the patient to develop a postoperative plan to control pain. Patients use patient-controlled analgesia pumps, an on-demand delivery of intravenous narcotics that patients control with a button release of a set dose of medication. The system has time lock-outs that are set by the provider to prevent the patient from administering too much medication. Nerve blocks and epidurals are used to prevent regional pain. A controlled dose of medication is managed by the anesthesia provider. Subcutaneous pain balls are placed to provide specific localized anesthetic to the patient and are commonly used at the donor skin sites after skin grafting is performed.

After a stay in the post anesthesia care unit (PACU), BPCU patients are continuously monitored 24 hours postoperatively with pulse oximetry. This monitoring is done to ensure that the patient's pain is well-managed without oversedation. Along with continuous monitoring of pulse oximetry, complete vital signs are obtained every 4 hours, and strict fluid and output monitoring is conducted.

Postoperative dressings remain in place for 3 to 8 days. The donor site dressing is removed after the first 24 hours to allow petroleum-impregnated gauze with antimicrobial properties to be placed on the site to dry and form a protective scab on the site. Graft sites are dressed based on size, extent, and physician preference and vary between negative-pressure wound dressings, silver-impregnated nylon dressings, and 5% Sulfamylon solution dressings. The nursing staff collaborate with rehabilitation staff to properly place splints on injured limbs and elevate them to protect the graft, avoid pressure points, and prevent contractures. Splints are also used to elevate arms to reduce edema. Leg nets, specially designed elevation devices with a pipe frame and elastic netting to create a hammocklike cradle, replace wedges and pillows for limb elevation. The primary function of the leg nets is to reduce edema and provide extra air circulation to donor sites that are wet or "soupy."

BPCU staff must remain vigilant as the patient recovers because of the large extent of open wounds, which increases the chance of electrolyte imbalance and hemodynamic instability caused by intraoperative blood and fluid loss. To facilitate healing, these patients continue with ongoing burn wound care including hydrotherapy and application of topical antimicrobial creams, solutions, or dressings in addition to excision and grafting surgeries. Intravenous and oral antibiotics are routinely ordered. Some BPCU nurses are trained for PACU recovery and will recover the BPCU patient in the PACU and return with them to the BPCU after recovery.[2]

DISCHARGE

The discharge portion of the patient's plan of care includes assessing and identifying current and anticipated psychosocial and physiologic needs, preparing and referring the patient for and to home health care or inpatient rehabilitation or to discharge home without additional services, and evaluating the effectiveness of self-care.[5] The patient's readiness for discharge is multifaceted. The components included in discharge planning assess the patients' and their family members' ability to leave an acute care facility. "Discharge readiness includes the patients' and families' perception of being prepared or not for hospital discharge."[5]

Several criteria must be met prior to discharge. The patient must be able to tolerate shower and wound care with oral pain medications and anxiolytics only. Patients must be able to perform their own wound care if they have no family or support available. Those who have family or a nonmedical attendant (NMA) available perform wound care with staff before discharge. The BPCU staff typically coordinate with the family or the NMA to have them start assisting with showers and wound care 4 to 6 days prior to anticipated discharge. This training helps the nurse determine the capabilities and willingness of the family member to properly care for the burns at home and reduces predischarge anxiety. Independence during showers and wound care is encouraged with nursing staff oversight. Family teaching for discharge allows the family member who will be helping the patient at home to feel comfortable with assisting the patient to bathe and apply dressings to the healing skin. If the caregiver is unable to adequately care for the patient or does not feel ready or comfortable, discharge is delayed until the person has the confidence to care for the patient independently.

Medications are reviewed with patient and caregiver prior to discharge. Staff question patients and family members about the medication regimen and discuss proper administration, which allows the nursing staff to screen for possible knowledge deficits to address before the patient goes home.[5] Multidisciplinary coordination with rehabilitation therapy, licensed providers, and case management allows nursing staff to facilitate discharge for the patient and family. The rehabilitation department schedules the patient for follow-up in their clinic during specific days throughout the week or that coincides with their follow-up clinic appointments. The rehabilitation department also provides printed home exercise instructions and teaches the patient and caregiver how and when to pressure-wrap extremities for edema control, which helps to minimize "tattooing," or blood pooling in the affected extremity while at home.

Included in the discharge teaching is the phone number for the BPCU so that the patient and family have a 24-hour number to call in case they have any questions about caring for themselves or their loved one. If a patient calls with a concern that cannot be resolved over the phone and they live in the area, staff will recommend that they return to the BPCU to be evaluated. If patients do not live in the area, they are instructed to seek care with their primary care provider or the local emergency department and to bring their discharge summary with them.

A follow up appointment is also scheduled for the patient in the burn clinic; the appointment is generally 4 to 7 days after discharge. The patient is discharged with enough medications to last until the follow-up appointment. Patients are instructed to call or return to the burn clinic if additional medications are needed. The patient is also provided with enough wound care supplies to last until their next appointment and some extra in case the dressings become soiled.

SUMMARY

The range of patient care varies in the BPCU from a patient directly admitted with a burn of less than 1% TBSA to those with original burns greater than 90% TBSA. Nurses in the BPCU must be intuitive when caring for patients and their families in order to accommodate the needs of each individual, ensure they receive quality inpatient care, and enable a smooth transition to the outpatient setting.

Caring for burn patients forms special bonds between burn center staff, the patient, and their family. This connection begins on admission and continues throughout the healing process, which may last for years. When a patient returns for follow-up outpatient appointments, he or she often comes back to the BPCU to visit the staff and to provide updates on their healing process, life at home, and family developments, and they bring the occasional home-baked goods!

A common catch phrase at the US Army Burn Center is "once a burn patient, always a burn patient." This patient population truly touches the hearts of those special nurses who care for them, and a unique bond is created between the nursing staff, the burn patient, and their loved ones that lasts for years.

REFERENCES

1. Saarmann L. Transfer out of critical care: freedom or fear? Crit Care Nurs Q 1993;16: 78–85.
2. Serio-Melvin M, Yoder LH, Gaylord KM. Caring for burn patients at the United States Institute for Surgical Research: the nurses' multifaceted roles. Nurs Clin North Am 2010;45:233–48.
3. Herndon DN. Total burn care. Galveston (TX): Saunders Elsevier; 2007.
4. Gilmartin J. Contemporary day surgery: patients' experience of discharge and recovery. J Clin Nurs 2007;16:1109–17.
5. Titler MG, Pettit DM. Discharge readiness assessment. J Cardiovasc Nurs 1995;9: 64–74.

Reconstructive Surgery in the Thermally Injured Patient

Davin Mellus, DMD[a],* Rodney K. Chan, MD[b]

KEYWORDS

- Microvascular free-tissue transfer • Pedicle flaps
- Reconstructive Surgery • Thermal injury • Z-plasties
- Skin grafting

AN INCREASED NEED FOR RECONSTRUCTIVE SURGERY

Reconstruction is a necessity in the complete care of the burn patient. This need has grown not only because of advances made in critical care resulting in improved patient survival, but also because of an increased number of burn admissions. In 2011, the American Burn Association approximated that 450,000 people suffer annually from burn injuries requiring medical treatment.[1] Of these, 45,000 require admission, 55% (24,750 admissions) will enter the 125 hospitals with specialized burn care centers,[2] an increase of 340% from 1995.[3] Among those admitted to these burn centers, the expected overall survival rate is 94.8%.[2] Depending on the depth and location of the burn injury, many of these patients require reconstructive surgery to ameliorate the late effect of burn scarring.

In addition to a greater demand for reconstruction secondary to the number of surviving patients, there has also been an increased awareness by patients and their providers that reconstructive surgery is a possibility. Furthermore, advances in tissue engineering and in surgical techniques have increased the options available to patients who previously might have "unreconstructable" deformities.

BASIC PHILOSOPHIES

The basic goal of all reconstruction is to restore form and function and to restore "like with like"; that is, replace tissue of a certain quality using other tissues of the same or

Conflicts of interest: The authors disclose no conflicts.

[a] Division of Oral and Maxillofacial Surgery, Dental and Trauma Research Detachment, United States Army Institute of Surgical Research, 3650 Chambers Pass, Fort Sam Houston, TX 78234, USA
[b] Division of Plastic and Reconstructive Surgery, Burn Scar Program, Dental and Trauma Research Detachment, Burn Center, United States Army Institute of Surgical Research, Brooke Army Medical Center, 3650 Chambers Pass, Fort Sam Houston, TX 78234, USA
* Corresponding author.
E-mail address: davin.mellus@us.army.mil

Perioperative Nursing Clinics 7 (2012) 107–113
doi:10.1016/j.cpen.2011.10.006
1556-7931/12/$ – see front matter Published by Elsevier Inc.

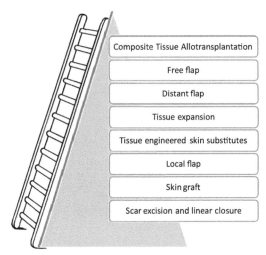

Fig. 1. Reconstructive ladder.

similar quality. Because burn scarring has functional, aesthetic, and psychosocial consequences,[4] burn reconstruction is among the most challenging reconstructive problems faced by plastic surgeons. Local tissues are often insufficient and scarred, vascular supply might have been compromised, and the tissues simply do not possess the normal characteristics we have come to know. Nevertheless, some basic guiding principles exist.

First, an accurate diagnosis of the deformity and an appraisal of the missing parts are essential. This step is particularly challenging in burn reconstruction because there is not often a physical deficit, at least not until an adequate excision or release has been performed. The "reconstructive ladder" (**Fig. 1**) is used as a guideline for the various available options, and often all rungs are needed in the management of severe deformities.[5] Realistic goals must be set from the start as to what might be achievable with the reconstruction. A thorough investigation into the history of the patient—in particular, the operations and flaps that were previously utilized and the available potential donor sites—is mandatory. Finally, it is important to formulate a comprehensive treatment plan based on the diagnosis. This plan is presented to the patient and his or her family with a timetable for reconstruction, emphasizing that the sequences are designed not to burn future bridges and that flexibility is necessary. A good rapport with the patient and his or her family is as important as the reconstructive plan. Rarely are 1 or 2 operations enough to achieve the result that the patient is looking for.

Burn scars change over time. In the first 3 years or even later, scars change in both color and quality. The characteristic redness and swelling of burn scars is more profound than that of traumatic wounds. For this reason, most reconstructive surgeons typically delay the reconstruction until 1 year or longer after the burn's occurrence to allow for inflammation to subside. Earlier reconstruction, although necessary at times, can result in less durable outcomes. Patients are informed that repeat releases might be necessary. However, there are clearly circumstances that dictate earlier surgical interventions, such as correction of ectropion to prevent exposure keratitis or correction of microstomia to improve dental hygiene and nutrition.[6]

Table 1					
Theoretic length increases with various Z-plasty angles					
Limb angle	30°	45°	60°	75°	90°
Gain in length (%)	25	50	75	100	120

Created with data from Hove C, Williams E, Rodgers B. Z-plasty: a concise review. Facial Plast Surg 2001;17:289–94.

Burn patients often do not remember their acute or reconstructive operations because of the heavy sedation utilized during much of their acute stay. In contrast, during later reconstructive procedures, not only are they cognizant of the multiple procedures required, but they are also invested in their own care. As a consequence, experienced perioperative burn nurses can be an excellent resource. In addition, even our best patients lose sight of the "big picture" at some point; encouragement from those experienced burn staff should always be seen as part of a curative treatment plan.

COMMON RECONSTRUCTIVE PROBLEMS AND TECHNIQUES

In burn reconstruction, 2 problems are rarely exactly alike. The unique distribution and depth of the thermal insult combined with each person's propensity to scarring makes each problem unique. However, there are some common themes. The head and neck and the extremities bear more than their share of the reconstructive burden. Full-thickness burn to the face and neck results in a stigmata that can include some or all of the following: Lower eyelid ectropion, short nose with ala flaring, short retruded upper lip, lower lip eversion, flat facial features, loss of jaw line definition, and lack of neck extension.[7] In the extremities, axillary, elbow, wrist, and webspace contractures are common. The specific choice of procedure and techniques varies depending on severity of the contracture and donor tissue availability. Some common techniques include Z-plasties, skin grafting, pedicle flaps, and microvascular free-tissue transfer.

Z-Plasty

The technique of a Z-plasty is composed of a central and 2 lateral incisions in a "Z" configuration. The lengths of the 3 limbs and angles formed between the primary and the secondary incisions are typically equal. This geometric rearrangement transforms the orientation and adds length to a contracted scar. Lengthening depends on the angles and configurations used. A classical Z-plasty uses 60° angles, granting a theoretical 75% increase in length (**Table 1**). Wider angles and longer limbs yield greater lengthening but require greater tissue mobility.[6] Flaps with an angle <45°, while easing closure, risk flap necrosis owing to decreased blood supply.[8] Typically, a Z-plasty is performed when a burn scar contracture is linear and there is adjacent tissue laxity. An example of multiple Z-plasties performed for release of an axillary contracture is shown in **Fig. 2**.

Full- and Split-Thickness Skin Grafting

As opposed to a Z-plasty, broad contractures often require transverse scar release or excision with tissue interposition. Often, the wound bed is sufficiently vascular after the release that a full-thickness skin graft or a split-thickness skin graft (STSG) can be applied. Although a full-thickness skin graft gives better esthetic appearance, an

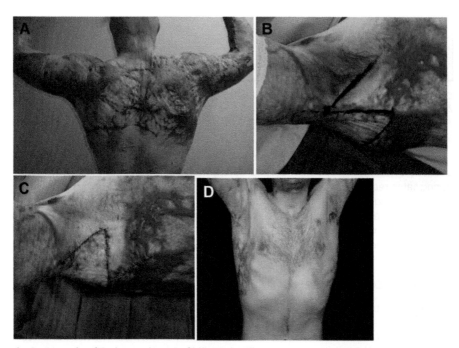

Fig. 2. Example of Z-plasty releases of bilateral axillary contractures. A 30-year-old man with truncal back and axillary burn scar contractures. He is unable to abduct his shoulders more than 90° degrees (*A*), a single Z-plasty was designed on the right (*B*), and 2 serial Z-plasties were designed on the left (not shown). The patient is shown immediately after flap transposition (*C*). Postoperative view is shown with near full abduction on the right and left abduction on the left (*D*).

STSG provides versatility, especially when large areas needing coverage are involved. When considering STSG donor sites, the upper posterolateral thigh is preferred; however, any available, healthy skin can theoretically be used. Consideration should be given to the concealablility of the donor scars as well as accessibility during surgery. In the case of a large burn and minimally available donor skin, options include repeat harvesting, meshing, and use of a dermal regeneration template with STSG. An STSG consists of the epidermis and dermis, typically anywhere from 8th to 16th/1000th of an inch. A thicker STSG can limit repeat harvests and can result in a problematic wound in children, the elderly, or other patients with thin, friable skin. Donor sites can generally be reharvested every 10 to 15 days, barring the presence of infection and depending on the initial depth. Disadvantages to the STSG correlate to its minimal dermal structure and include the tendency for recurrent contractures. full-thickness skin graft s are usually reserved for reconstructions with functional (hands or neck) or aesthetic (eyelids, perioral) areas. The required donor site must have redundant skin; and typically the supraclavicular, lateral thoracic, lower abdominal, or groin areas are chosen. Since harvesting includes removal of all regenerative dermal layers down to adipose tissue, the donor site should ideally retain enough laxity for a primary closure. Although an FTSG provides more cutaneous biology and generally better aesthetics, the graft survival rate is lower than for an STSG; and wound preparation is paramount.[9] An example of broad back contracture released by using an STSG is shown **Fig. 3**.

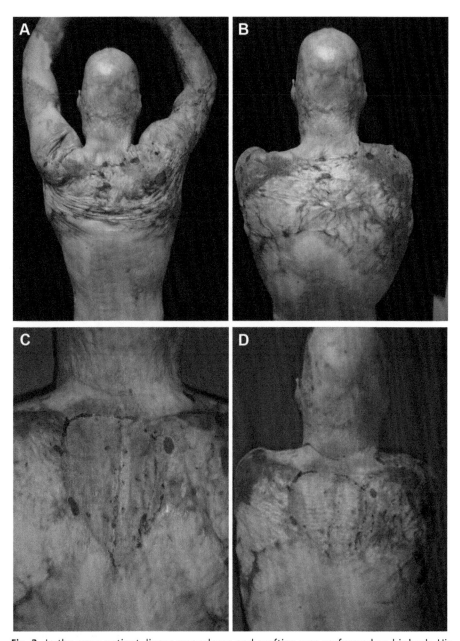

Fig. 3. In the same patient, linear scar release and grafting was performed on his back. His back contracture limits shoulder abduction despite correction of axillary contractures (*A*). Shoulder extension similarly results in recurring stress–relaxation of the scar (*B*). Linear contracture release without scar excision followed by grafting led to improvement of the tightness (*C*), especially with shoulder extension (*D*).

Pedicled and Free-Flap Closures

Flaps are chosen over grafts when the underlying wound bed cannot support a graft or when the possibility of recontracture not tolerated. Skin flaps are not vascularized by the wound bed, but carry their own blood supply. For that reason, they can be used to cover areas where graft loss is common because of movement or poor vascularity.[10] Local flaps are from adjacent areas, whereas distant flaps come from nonadjacent areas. A free microvascular flap, a type of a distant flap, involves microanastomoses of the donor and recipient arteries and veins. Flaps are very useful in burn resurfacing, but do have the disadvantages of being very bulky and often require additional revisional operations.

UNIQUE PERIOPERATIVE CONSIDERATIONS
Preoperative

An integrated approach to caring for a burn patient is of utmost importance. Facial scarring is incredibly visible and psychologically traumatic, creating some unique problems in providing care. The process must be flexible, and surgical plans can change, even preoperatively and sometimes intraoperatively. Because there is not often a single complete "fix," families and patients need reassurance from the burn team that although the process may require multiple operations and the course of treatment will very likely change with each procedure and its results, each operation moves toward the ultimate goal.[11] For patients undergoing autografts or flap transfers, preoperative education and discussion minimizes the unpleasantness of receiving yet another wound. Incorporating frequent updates helps to reduce the emotional turmoil inherent in reconstructive procedures.

Intraoperative

The duration of reconstructive operations varies depending on the selected procedure. Even with releases with or without grafting, reconstructive operations can become lengthy when performed on multiple sites. An appropriate amount of time must be taken to ensure the best possible outcome, especially when working with valuable and often limited donor tissue. Ensuring appropriate management of body temperature and fluids during the course of a prolonged operation is essential and can be significantly more complicated, even in burn reconstruction patients. In addition to the typical surgical concerns of padding, eye protection, and deep vein thrombosis prophylaxis, consideration and attention must be given to the increased possibility of positional changes and diminished quantities of soft tissue. Airway concerns must consider prior inhalation injury, late nasal or tracheal stenosis, and the possible addition of neck contracture and microstomia restricting airway access.

Postoperative

As with every step of the process, good communication is essential among staff members. Discussion with the operative team, patient, and family regarding procedures performed and postoperative care helps to ensure compliance and reconstructive success. Immobilization and rehabilitation after grafting are often crucial for success, but must be balanced between graft incorporation and prevention of joint contractures.[12]

SUMMARY

Although the operations required during acute burn hospitalization are life-saving, subsequent reconstructive operations can be life-giving. Each reconstructive plan is tailored for each patient, depending on the specific deformity. Multiple reconstructive modalities are possible, but the goal is always restoration of form and function. The operative plan must include preoperative, intraoperative, and postoperative considerations to be successful.

ACKNOWLEDGMENTS
The opinions or assertions contained herein are the private views of the authors and are not to be construed as official or as reflecting the views of the Department of the Army or the Department of Defense.

REFERENCES

1. National Hospital Ambulatory Medical Care Survey (NHAMCS); National Ambulatory Medical Care Survey (NAMC); National Electronic Injury Surveillance System-All Injury Project (NEISS-AIP). 2008 data.
2. American Burn Association. National Burn Repository. 2010.
3. American Burn Association. National Burn Repository. 2006.
4. Shelley OP, Dziewulski P. Late management of burns. Surgery Oxford 2006;24:15.
5. Boyce DE, Shokrollahi K. Reconstructive surgery. BMJ 2006;332:710–12.
6. Hudson DA. Some thoughts on choosing a Z-plasty: the Z made simple. Plast Reconstr Surg 2000;106:665.
7. Donelan, MB. In: Thorne C, Beasley R, Aston S, et al, editors. Grabb and Smith's plastic surgery. 6th edition. Philadelphia: Kluwer; 2007. p. 150–61.
8. Furnas DW, Fischer GW. The Z-plasty: biomechanics and mathematics. Br J Plast Surg 1971;24:144.
9. Adams DC, Ramsey ML. Grafts in dermatologic surgery: review and update on full- and split thickness skin grafts, free cartilage grafts, and composite grafts. Dermatol Surg 2005;31:1055.
10. Huang T. Overview of burn reconstruction. In: Herndon D, editor. Total burn care. 3rd edition. Philadelphia: WB Saunders; 2007. p. 674.
11. Coleman JJ. Achauer and Sood's burn surgery: reconstruction and rehabilitation. Philadelphia: Saunders; 2006. p. 1.
12. Connor-Ballard PA. Understanding and managing burn pain: part 1. Am J Nursing 2009;109:4.

Trauma-Induced Coagulopathy: An Update to Current Management

Christopher V. Maani, MD, MC, US Army[a],*, Peter A. DeSocio, DO[b]

KEYWORDS

- Coagulopathy • Management • Resuscitation • Trauma

Key points

- In patients with hemorrhagic shock, clinicians must anticipate and manage the coagulopathy of trauma closest to onset of injury as possible.
- Untreated coagulopathy of trauma increases likelihood a patient will develop hemorrhagic shock and multiorgan system failure.
- Hemostatic transfusion strategies focused on early and liberal use of plasma, platelets, cryoprecipitate and coagulation factor isolates result in decreased blood loss in trauma patients.
- Point-of-care testing, thromboelastography, coagulation panels, lactate and local PO2 can identify problems sooner and manage coagulopathies efficiently for improved outcomes.

Advances in military and civilian prehospital care and evacuation, while centered around reduction in morbidity and mortality, have left trauma specialists facing new challenges in the areas of post injury resuscitation and in the treatment of trauma induced coagulopathies. Increased survival of patients from the point of injury to trauma centers for definitive medical treatment has forced a change in the way we medically manage modern day casualties. Evolving recommendations on the best practice of trauma resuscitation continues to change landscape of medical centers all around the globe. With the advent of new noninvasive medical devices along with

---

The opinions expressed herein are those of the authors and are not to be construed as official or reflecting the views of the US Department of Defense.

The authors have nothing to disclose.

[a] Department of Anesthesiology, United States Army Institute of Surgical Research and Army Burn Center, Brooke Army Medical Center, 3400 Rawley East Chambers Avenue, Fort Sam Houston, TX 78234, USA

[b] Department of Anesthesiology, The Ohio State University Medical Center, 410 West 10th Avenue, Columbus, OH 43210, USA

* Corresponding author.

E-mail address: Christopher.Maani@us.army.mil

rapid point-of-care testing in thromboelastography (TEG), coagulation panels, lactate, and local Po_2, there is the potential to improve patient outcomes by allowing for quicker triaging and transfer times of multiple casualties from onset of injury to frontline trauma physicians for treatment. These laboratory and technological advances may directly improve patient outcomes by recognizing true emergencies earlier and referral for surgical interventions sooner. Although once it was thought that mortality was summarily independent of medical interventions and resuscitations, we now know the opposite to be true; it is our expectation and indeed our obligation to recognize and manage the coagulopathy of trauma better than in past years. The worldwide medical community continues to struggle and debate the best course of action to reduce the leading cause of preventable death, which is massive hemorrhage. Inasmuch as we continue to improve in our management of trauma resuscitation and strive to prevent acidosis, hypothermia, and the progressive coagulopathy following injury, there is still much work to be done through evidence-based medicine, research, and new device technologies to demonstrate improved survival rates in trauma victims who require massive transfusion. Continued research efforts are still under way around the world to convert many of the controversies in management of coagulopathy and resuscitation into standardization of practice for physicians.

HISTORICAL PERSPECTIVE

Throughout history, major advancements in military and civilian medicine have occurred during conflict while treating injuries sustained by our wounded warriors. Visionaries who formed the first mobile hospitals, trained the first field medics, or developed the first air medical evacuation via the helicopter should be acknowledged for helping shape the landscape of our current military and civilian trauma systems. Our present medical transport evacuations, along with the use of new medical tourniquets, are just a few of the advances in trauma medicine that have helped prevent exsanguination from extremity injuries. The concept of hemorrhage control taught to medical specialists in both the military and civilian training programs has allowed today's trauma victims to reach medical treatment facilities for definitive treatment sooner and in more stable condition than was previously possible.

The idea that a certain percentage of deaths are preventable is not a new perception made by trauma specialists. In fact, throughout history it is easy to find documentation observing the death of a man secondary to uncontrolled bleeding. COL H.M. Gray in 1919 stated that "The hemorrhage that takes place when a main artery is divided is usually so rapid and so copious that the wounded man dies before help can reach him".[1] It is somewhat surprising that today we continue to struggle with the problem of potentially preventable morbidity and mortality seen decades ago that stem from inadequate control of hemorrhage and coagulopathy, often developed at the time of injury to the initiation definitive treatment by physicians. In fact, despite all current advances in the evacuation chain, pharmaceutical development, and medical devices for treatment and recognition of uncontrolled bleeding; massive hemorrhage in US soldiers (engaged in combat) continues to account for over one-third of trauma-related deaths. In addition hemorrhage is the leading cause of potentially preventable deaths following major trauma.[2–4] The study[3] details the incidence, causative mechanisms and effects of traumatic hemorrhage, both domestic and international. Hemorrhage ranks second in overall causes of prehospital deaths according to Tieu and colleagues.[5] Massive hemorrhage in major trauma victims correlates to high mortality in the early postoperative period.[6] Whether it is a combat medic on the battlefield, a civilian paramedic in the prehospital environment, or a trauma physician in a tertiary care center, understanding the principles of early resuscitative treatment for massive hemorrhage and avoiding complications related to early trauma coagulopathies could lead to improved patient outcomes and decreased mortality.

A small number of trauma patients who arrive to the emergency department are in a hypocoaguable state, and it is this minority that accounts for 50% of the blood product usage and the majority of in-hospital trauma-related deaths. Recent studies also show that coagulopathy starts early following trauma and that massive transfusion is associated with increased risk of death.[7] Currently, there are 2 likely theories behind early trauma-induced coagulopathy. One hypothesis involves the development of a disseminated intravascular coagulopathy–like pattern with altered fibrinolysis secondary to tissue factor generation and increased thrombin formation, and the second comprises tissue hypoperfusion leading to activated protein C and ultimately systemic anticoagulation.[8] Perioperative and emergency medicine literature describe the concept of trauma damage control for reducing hemorrhage and prevention of hemorrhagic shock to improve morbidity and mortality outcomes.[4,9,10] A new concept of "damage control resuscitation" has emerged that addresses the entire triad of death on admission to medical treatment facilities and calls into question how soon coagulation factor replacement should be used in early active hemorrhage following trauma.[11–13]

Military experts have also used damage control resuscitation during the current wars in Iraq and Afghanistan to decrease long-term mortality through early diagnosis and treatment of hemorrhage and hypovolemic shock.[7] While traditional practices to treat hemorrhage have focused efforts solely on treating hypotension, acidosis, and hypothermia plus achieving surgical control of bleeding, new research supports the practice of preventing coagulopathy in early stages of trauma. Current opinion by military and civilian experts backed by recent literature from current global conflicts supports the addition of coagulopathy as a primary focus in the treatment of patients with traumatic hemorrhage. While traditional practices are suitable for most trauma patients, these practices are often not appropriate for that subset of patients who are in hemorrhagic shock.[7] Although previously calling for immediate and aggressive intravenous fluid resuscitation of patients in hemorrhagic shock, current guidelines in Advanced Trauma Life Support have been revised to direct care toward managing controllable hemorrhage and leaning toward a more hemostatic goal for the resuscitation rather than just prevention of hypotension and circulatory collapse.[11,14,15] The study[14] demonstrated yet another reason to aggressively pursue normothermia. Temperature alterations disrupt the coagulation cascade by inhibition of the effects of von Willebrand factor (vWF).

The conventional approach of immediate volume resuscitation with 2:1 isotonic crystalloids and plasma-poor red blood cells (RBCs) to manage early active hemorrhage is often counterproductive and may potentiate hypothermia, acidosis, and progressive coagulopathy, commonly referred to as the "lethal triad of death." Even though these unbalanced resuscitative efforts may promote oxygen delivery and tissue perfusion; RBCs and crystalloid and colloid solutions often carry the potential to destabilize the patient's tenuous condition following trauma. The reasoning behind this theory is that massive fluid administration can disrupt the electrolyte balance, further dilute coagulation factors, and impair clot formation, which can result in greater transfusion requirements. Periods of massive colloid or crystalloid resuscitation owing to periods of raised blood pressure has been referred to as the "pop the clot" phenomenon.[16] In fact, following the development of the lethal triad, Cosgriff and colleagues[15] have shown that the sum and severity of these components along with injury severity can account for the incidence of coagulopathy approaching 100%

and mortality reaching almost 60%. To address these issues, most damage control resuscitation protocols consist of limiting resuscitation volume to protect newly formed clot. Preliminary results in a recent human prospective randomized control trial suggest that hypotensive resuscitation strategies are safe and show less severe coagulopathies, while improving overall mortality in early postoperative period.[17] Although these findings are not without their limitations, it is the first study to address the efficacy of deliberate hypotensive resuscitation in human subjects. Restoring intravascular volume directed at normalizing international normalized ratio, base deficit, dilutional thrombocytopenia, and low fibrinogen levels are goals that should be achieved in a rapid and efficient manner. The trend of most trauma centers around the world is to develop massive transfusion protocols that consist of a fresh frozen plasma–to–packed RBC a ratio of 1:1, platelets, and cryoprecipitate to address in a standardized approach toward dealing with coagulopathy sooner during massive hemorrhage.

OBJECTIVES

Following combat-related injury or civilian trauma, the anesthesiologist, surgeon, intensivist, and emergency medicine physician must all work in conjunction as a team to control bleeding and prevent exsanguination. Although management of hemorrhage control and resuscitation efforts start preoperatively and as close to the onset of injury as possible, damage control strategies must continue during the intraoperative and postoperative periods for maximum patient benefit. Treating life-threatening uncontrollable bleeding, whether due to vascular injury or gross coagulopathy, requires a multidisciplinary approach to include surgical interventions (ie, suture ligation and electrocautery) and resuscitative efforts focused on directing blood component therapy to optimally achieve hemostasis.[10] The keys to decreased morbidity and mortality following trauma can be realized through focused understanding of coagulopathy in trauma patients, along with appreciating the physiologic and environmental factors that influence its severity. These coagulopathic concerns start immediately after acute trauma in which fibrinolysis and release of D-dimers are detected within 30 minutes of injury and continue throughout the perioperative course.[4,18,19]

In this review, we discuss the factors that influence the coagulopathy of trauma and how each component affects patient outcomes and clinical decision-making. In addition, we briefly address diagnosis, treatment, and management strategies to proactively limit the complications and sequelae associated with the lethal triad of death.

Factors Affecting the Coagulopathy in Trauma Patients

The body's intrinsic hemostatic regulatory mechanisms involve a principal balance between clot formation and breakdown. Following endothelial injury, clot initiation occurs through vasoconstriction, platelet plug creation, fibrin mesh formation, and lysis.[3] Factors that influence the coagulopathy of trauma can also be divided into 4 main groups: hypothermia, acidosis, complications of resuscitation, and additional factors.

Hypothermia

Multiple etiologies that predispose a patient to hypothermia following major trauma include, but are not limited to, fluid and blood product administration, environmental exposure, and hemorrhagic shock.[20] Even though hypothermia is used as a technique to protect against end organ failure and ischemia, there is no indication following hemorrhagic shock and ongoing hemorrhage. Hypothermia (accidental or exposure hypothermia is defined as core body temperature of <35°C and severe hypothermia as core temperature <32°C) is a key factor in the coagulopathy after trauma and uncontrolled bleeding in the operating room.[3,9,18,21–24] Hypothermia is an independent risk factor following trauma, and mortality rates increase the greater the drop in core body temperature from normothermia.[20] In fact, one prospective observational study looking at prehospital core body temperature in major trauma victims reports a 3-fold increase in risk of death when prehospital hypothermia (<35°C) occurs.[25] Martini and colleagues[24] studied the isolated effects of these procoagulopathic conditions in situ using a porcine model. The American Society of Anesthesiology (ASA) recognized the importance of monitoring temperature for management of hypothermia when it issued the ASA standard for temperature monitoring; this is the recommendation that "every patient receiving anesthesia shall have temperature monitored when clinically significant changes in body temperature are intended, anticipated or suspected."[26] The study[26] was among the first to stress the importance and need for intraoperative temperature monitoring and management. Hypothermia either following trauma or present intraoperatively is secondary to one of the 4 mechanisms of heat loss: conduction, convection, radiation, and evaporation. Addressing these mechanisms may assist in the maintenance of normothermia and prevention of the development of hypothermia, which is all too often detrimental in the case of the bleeding trauma patient. Prevention of hypothermia should not be overlooked as an important management strategy following trauma. Not only has medical literature shown decreases in mortality rates with normothermia, but also there is evidence to suggest that there are decreases in hemorrhage, fluid requirements, multisystem organ failure, and length in intensive care unit stays, when hypothermia is prevented.[20] A recent study by Dirkmann and colleagues[9] demonstrated impaired stability of clots as well as slowed initiation and propagation of coagulation during periods of hypothermia. Specifically, hypothermia affects platelet activation and adhesion at the molecular level by inhibiting the interaction of vWF and platelet glycoprotein Ib–IX–V complex.[16] When patients lack adequate compensatory thermoregulatory mechanisms required to maintain normothermia in response to cold stressors, avoidance of hypothermia to prevent coagulopathy is an important practice strategy.[18,21,23]

In addition to the heat loss associated with trauma and the prehospital phase, intraoperative heat loss during initiation and maintenance of general anesthesia results initially in a rapid decrease in core temperature followed by a linear reduction in core temperature; this is discussed in a chapter taken from Miller's *Anesthesia*,[27] the most commonly accepted "bible" of anesthesia texts. This characteristic anesthesia-induced pattern of hypothermia is compounded by rapid intravascular volume expansion with relatively cold intravenous fluids or blood components during rapid administration of resuscitative products in the face of continued operative or traumatic hemorrhage. The hypothermic insult is associated with a decrease in thrombin generation as well as compromised formation of both platelet plugs and fibrin clots.[15,24] In addition to the qualitative platelet deficit, there is an increase in lysis of clots.

Acidosis

Usually characterized by an acidemic pH of less than 7.35, acidosis also has profound effects on coagulopathy following trauma and often is the result of, but not limited to, the administration of large fluid resuscitations with supraphysiologic concentrations of chloride relative to sodium.[28,29] In fact, metabolic acidosis probably plays a bigger role on inhibiting coagulation than does hypothermia. Martini and colleagues report that the effects of pH neutralization following acidosis on the reversibility of coagulopathy in vivo or in vitro studies are prolonged compared to rapid correction of coagulopathy from hypothermia following rewarming. These findings suggest that acidosis, due to a nonreversible effect on coagulation, is more harmful to the coagulation profile of trauma patients.[30] A common strategy for treating acute hypotension in the operating room or during first response in field medicine is the bolus administration of crystalloid solutions. Although isotonic saline is often chosen, balanced crystalloid solutions such as Ringer's lactate solution are also common. Even after assuming an intact Cori cycle and the absence of shock liver, lactate can impose an acid load that is poorly tolerated by physiologic buffer systems that are already compromised.[31] This has led some researchers to examine buffers as mediators to improve the coagulopathy of trauma, although results have not been inspiring.[32]

Recent studies have demonstrated that acidosis alone can worsen coagulopathy by inhibiting the enzyme complexes that are vital to thrombin formation, a factor required for conversion of fibrinogen to fibrin and the activation of other cofactors essential for hemostasis. The combination of acidosis and hypothermia can lead to severe coagulopathy and disastrous consequences. Dirkmann and colleagues[9] showed a synergistic effect on impairment of coagulation when acidosis was added to existing hypothermia but failed to show a significant change in all viscoelastic properties of clot formation (except clot lysis) when studying acidosis alone. In addition, the severity of acidosis and hypothermia in this study showed more impairment in coagulation parameters than the mathematical sum of each. Martini and colelagues[24] showed increased bleeding time and thrombin generation when severe acidosis and hypothermia were combined in a swine model.

Complications of resuscitation and transfusion therapy

The perfusion insult and acidosis seen after trauma are worsened by the commonly used blood preservative citrate phosphate dextrose (with adenine or adenine, dextrose, sorbitol, sodium chloride, and mannitol) and by old blood.[33,34] Citrate phosphate dextrose and citrate phosphate dextrose adenine solutions are often responsible for low levels of 2,3-diphosphoglyceric acid. The longer the blood is banked (especially after 21 days), the greater the acidosis seen in conjunction with CO_2 accumulation and buildup of acids as byproducts of RBC metabolism.[13,33] The resulting left shift in the hemoglobin (Hb)–O_2-carrying curve means decreased oxygen release from Hb. Although outcomes related to blood product administration could be multifactorial, retrospective data looking at RBC transfusion alone may be linked to increased mortality and morbidity, primarily in acute respiratory distress syndrome and multisystem organ failure. It is no surprise that retrospective studies have found an association of increased morbidity and mortality with the use of older RBC products (>14 days of storage) versus the use of fresh RBC products (<14 days of storage).[8] A dilutional coagulopathy, seen during initial and ongoing resuscitations with fluids such as crystalloids and packed RBCs, which are poor in clotting factors, is the unwanted byproduct of focusing on restoration of intravascular volume rather than hemostasis.[13,35] In doing so, well meaning but ill-informed clinicians provide fodder for the adage "drive the pressure and pop the clot." Once translated, the study[35] offers a compelling argument for deliberate hypotensive resuscitation of a bleeding trauma patient. As discussed previously, hypothermia can, in and of itself, cause tremendous dysfunction within the coagulation cascade. Cold storage requirements for erythrocytes, plasma, and cryoprecipitate compound the sting of trauma coagulopathy by leading to qualitative platelet defects and impaired coagulation enzyme pathways when normothermia is compromised after transfusion. When these functional defects are considered along with the acidic milieu of a typical 21-day-old unit of RBCs with pH often approximating 6.3, it is clear that RBC transfusion is no magic bullet.[33,36]

Additional factors

In addition to acidosis, hypothermia, and hemodilution, several additional factors are implicated in the coagulopathy of trauma. Although often unmentioned, hemorrhage and extravasation of clotting factors are as detrimental as the consumption of platelets and coagulation factors, often referred to as consumption coagulopathy.[10] Increased fibrinolysis is associated with hypothermia, anoxia, perfusion deficits, and tissue damage.[15,37] The overall pattern of fibrinolysis in the trauma population is particularly puzzling as both hyperfibrinolytic and hypofibrinolytic states have been encountered.[38] Point-of-care TEG and coagulation function tests demonstrate their merits in these circumstances, whereas laboratory-based routine coagulation panels understate the coagulopathy as they are assayed at 37°C and often require 30 to 60 minutes to provide a result. Several other causes have also been identified in the altered coagulatory profile of trauma patients. Detrimental effects of colloids such as hetastarches, in doses of greater than 20 mL/kg per day, are believed to impair the coagulatory profile as well.[3] Both hemodilution and platelet impairment are implicated when these resuscitative fluids are chosen to replete intravascular volume. Because ionized calcium is required for normal clotting, hypocalcemia often leads to deficits in the clotting cascade.[39] The clinical course following severe trauma often resembles disseminated intravascular coagulation, with similar findings such as multiple intravascular clots and discrete necrotic lesions.[40]

Monitoring

A high index of suspicion is essential when identifying a patient that requires massive transfusion in order to implement early definitive treatment and improved outcomes. Unfortunately, when signs of shock develop (ie, hypotension and tachycardia) in a trauma patients, resuscitation efforts are often delayed. There is evidence to suggest that using specific indices may help identify patients at risk for massive transfusion. Using a simple ratio of heart rate to systolic blood pressure to calculate the shock index, medical providers can assess risk of massive transfusion for acute trauma. The shock index has the potential to recognize hemorrhage not always evident by visual examination (ie, blunt abdominal trauma).[41] In addition, there are new medical devices that can measure continuous hemoglobin noninvasively and have promise in triaging trauma casualties.

Traditionally, when blood products and fluids are administered during ongoing surgical bleeding, physicians have had to rely on monitoring frequent serial laboratory test results such as prothrombin time, activated partial thromboplastin time, platelet count, blood fibrinogen levels, and fibrin degradation products.[37,42] These results may be used to guide transfusion requirements and improve coagulation profiles.[43] Clinically, however, this is not the case because from the time coagulation samples are sent for laboratory analysis to the time results are available, 30 to 60 minutes may routinely pass. This is sufficient time for the clinical picture to completely change and deteriorate for victims of severe trauma. Although the duration of obtaining laboratory results is standard, the utility of these relatively delayed results for clinical decision-making is limited because of the constant change in coagulation profile during ongoing resuscitative efforts. Point-of-care TEG and coagulation function tests demonstrate their merits in these circumstances, whereas laboratory-based routine coagulation panels are not time-sensitive nor do they accurately reflect the coagulopathy coincident with hypothermia as they are assayed at 37°C.[44] Clinically relevant laboratory information that may affect a physician's decision to treat a specific form of coagulopathy in the trauma patient requires rapid acquisition and quantification of the coagulation process as a whole. TEG provides a dynamic and graphic qualitative depiction of the coagulation capacity based on viscoelastic properties of blood, and it also provides quantitative information based on clot initiation and maturation. TEG determines the time for initial fibrin formation, the rate of fibrin deposition, clot consistency, the rate of clot formation, and lysis.[43] However, operation and analysis of TEG data often require clinicians and laboratory personnel with experience in interpreting TEG graphs. Familiarity and experience with clinical TEGs can be very beneficial when it comes to guiding the choice of resuscitative fluids and directing blood component therapy.[45,46]

TREATMENTS

This is an age of limited resources due in part to ongoing global conflicts, rising health care costs and reform, and the increasing demand for evidence-based medicine. Novel, safe, and cost-effective treatments for the management of coagulopthy of trauma are being investigated as replacement for traditional standard practice. Although recognition of the factors implicated in the coagulopathy of trauma are important, the prevention and management of this coagulopathy are paramount to improving outcomes. Even though there is conflicting literature regarding the approach to best practice methods for the treatment of trauma-associated coagulopathy, recent trends in research that demonstrate potential benefit have focused on increased predetermined ratios of plasma to erythrocytes, increased use of cryoprecipitate, platelets, recombinant factor VIIa (rFVIIa), human fibrinogen extracts, desmopressin acetate (DDAVP), and conjugated estrogens.[18,28] In traditional resuscitation, guidelines often require the administration of large volumes of crystalloids intravenously, which we are realizing today can compound the coagulation defect and lead to undesired outcomes such as abdominal compartment syndrome, pulmonary edema, airway edema, and cardiovascular sequelae. However, early aggressive use of plasma, platelets, and cryoprecipitate combined with component-directed transfusion therapy driven by TEG can improve short-term considerations such as cumulative transfusion requirements as well as long-term outcomes such as survival.[11,47] Although the debate continues over the need and the likelihood of large multicenter prospective randomized clinical trials investigating the role of rFVIIa, fresh whole blood, and lyophilized blood products such as plasma and platelets in the management of marked coagulopathy of trauma, new studies show promise in safety and efficacy. As clinicians, it is recommended that we rely on our own clinical judgments and relevant studies available to guide our damage control resuscitation and correction of trauma coagulopathy.[12,48,49]

A major priority for military physicians and researchers when considering the utilization of new medical products and devices is the reduction in the logistical footprint on both the battlefield and prehospital austere environments. In addition, a major objective is to address the current problems faced when practicing medicine in these types of remote locations, such as storage and expiration of products used to treat coagulopathy of trauma, which are often obstacles to successful treatment of active hemorrhage. All too often these potential breakthroughs in trauma medicine are in the early stages of research and development and cannot be marketed for patient use until evidence proving benefit and no harm has been studied. Some hemostatic agents and dressings used to prevent and treat the coagulopathy of trauma currently fall into this category. Development and testing are under way using different forms of dried plasma as a source of concentrated clotting factors. In fact, early animal studies using spray-dried plasma show that clotting factors are preserved using this method and that this product is shelf-stable and low-volume and demonstrates similar effectiveness in reversing trauma-associated coagulopathy compared to standard fresh frozen plasma administration.[50] If results are consistent in human subjects, this alternative plasma replacement has the potential to be an excellent treatment option when faced with scarce resources in an austere combat environment.

The effect of tranexamic acid on mortality resulting from acute trauma bleeding has also been investigated as a novel pharmacologic treatment for the control of traumatic hemorrhage. Acute coagulopathy differs from other mechanisms of coagulopathy (ie, hemodilution, hypothermia, or acidosis) by virtue of the physiologic pathway of acute trauma. There seems to be evidence to suggest that acute coagulopathy and hemorrhage increase the systemic byproducts of fibrinolysis (D-dimers) shortly after shock or tissue injury. Therefore, an antifibrinolyitic pharmacologic agent, like tranexamic acid, should be able to prevent complete activation of fibrinolysis.[19] Recent analysis by the collaborators of the CRASH-2 randomized control trial suggest that there is an improved survival rate in patients receiving tranexamic acid up to 3 hours post injury.[51] Although these results are promising, improved mortality is also linked to the time of administration of transexamic acid and onset of injury. Investigators of this study suggest an increase in mortality if patients receive treatment greater than 3 hours post injury. Although the exact mechanisms for this finding are unclear, investigators theorize that the increased mortality could be due to disseminated intravascular coagulation (a late finding in trauma) or to the formation of a prothrombin occurs earlier after trauma or be the result of patients who arrive later for definitive treatment who may have already developed physiologic signs of the classic "lethal triad of death."

Even though the potential for new developments in medical products used for resuscitation are limitless, the jury is still out on the efficacy and safety of many of these treatment options for the uncontrolled bleeding patient and the prevention of coagulation of trauma. In addition, there is currently no substitute for use of approved tourniquets and topical hemostatic agents that help stem active hemorrhage and reduce the need for further dilution of clotting factors with fluids other than fresh whole blood.[2,4,13,52] This goes hand in hand with deliberate limitation of hetastarch and colloids associated with aggravated hemodilution and impaired coagulatory profiles.[2,3] In decreasing actual blood loss, native clotting factors will remain in situ, whereas hemostatic ground is gained most easily.[36,53]

Not forgetting the importance of environment factors influencing coagulopathy, treatments focused on maintaining normothermia are vital to successful hemostasis following trauma. Aggressive use of fluid warmers, heated trauma operative suites, and temperature conservation technologies to include intravascular temperature management catheters and surface warming applications, are indicated to minimize detrimental physiologic effects hypothermia has on patients after injury.[23,28] New technologies including circulating water warmers and countercurrent heat exchange systems are on the horizon to address the challenges encountered when dealing with temperature management following major trauma.[20] The prevention and treatment of acidosis must be stressed throughout the hospital course, and perfusion deficits must be limited to minimize lactic acidosis.[10] Along with frequent monitoring of acid-base status, clinicians must stay vigilant to ward off the acute hypocalcemia so common after transfusion with citrate-rich blood products.[5] A key player in the coagulation cascade as factor IV, ionized calcium should be monitored throughout the resuscitation to avoid the pitfalls of hypocalcemia, which, through vigilant monitoring, is readily corrected. Acute hypocalcemia of trauma is most often secondary to either citrate toxicity or hypothermia.[54]

SUMMARY

Trauma resuscitation paradigms have changed in military and civilian medical centers over the past decade from large crystalloid administration to early blood component therapy using massive transfusion protocols. Although the coagulation defects following severe trauma may not be completely reversible, the dividends are great for any improvement toward hemostasis. While hemorrhage-control strategies such as extremity tourniquet use, deliberate hypotension, and damage control resuscitation must be used as first-line treatments following trauma, consideration should be given toward the addition of rFVIIa, DDAVP, conjugated estrogens, and lyophilized blood products to a clinician's armamentarium to combat traumatic hemorrhage. Revised transfusion ratios call for early and more aggressive use of plasma and fibrinogen-rich blood products, including fresh whole blood for emergency use in severe hemorrhage and massive transfusion. If addressed early after the onset of injury, coagulopathy of trauma is laden with opportunities for clinicians to intervene by treating the factors responsible for the deficit: acidosis, hypothermia, progressive coagulopathy, hypocalcemia, consumption, and hyperfibrinolysis. Aggressive monitoring, early management, and fundamental avoidance of these factors are critical in improving patient outcomes following trauma.

REFERENCES

1. Hemorrhage control. In: Burris DG, Dougherty PJ, Elliot DC, FitzHarris JB, et al, editors. Emergency war surgery. 3rd US revision. Washington, DC: Office of the Surgeon General, Borden Institute; 2004. p. 6.1.
2. Holcomb JB. Methods for improved hemorrhage control. Crit Care 2004;8:S57–60.
3. Kauvar DS, Wade CE. The epidemiology and modern management of traumatic hemorrhage: US and international perspectives. Crit Care 2005;9(Suppl 5): S1–9.
4. Eastridge BJ, Malone D, Holcomb JB. Early predictors of transfusion and mortality after injury: a review of the data-based literature. J Trauma 2006;60:S20–5.
5. Tieu BH, Holcomb JB, Schreiber MA. Coagulopathy: its pathophysiology and treatment in the injured patient. World J Surg 2007;31:1055–64.
6. Hoyt DB, Bulger EM, Knudson MM, et al. Death in the operating room: an analysis of a multicenter experience. J Trauma 1994;37:426–32.
7. Holcomb JB. Damage control resuscitation. In: Nessen SC, Lounsbury DE, Hetz SP, editors. War surgery in Afghanistan and Iraq: a series of cases, 2003-2007. 1st edition. Washington, DC: Office of The Surgeon General, Borden Institute, Walter Reed Army Medical Center; 2008. p. 49–51.
8. Shaz BH, Dente CJ, Harris JB, et al. Transfusion management in trauma patients. Anesth Analg 2009;108:1760–8.
9. Dirkmann D, Hanke AA, Gorlinger K, et al. Hypothermia and acidosis synergistically impair coagulation in human whole blood. Anesth Analg 2008;106:1627–32.
10. Rossaint R, Cerny V, Coats TJ, et al. Key issues in advanced bleeding care in trauma. Shock 2006;26:322–31.

11. Hess JR, Holcomb JB, Hoyt DB. Damage control resuscitation: the need for specific blood products to treat the coagulopathy of trauma. Transfusion 2006; 46:685–6.

12. Mittermayr M, Streif W, Haas T, et al. Hemostatic changes after crystalloid or colloid fluid administration during major orthopedic surgery: the role of fibrinogen administration. Anesth Analg 2007;105:905–17.

13. Spinella PC. Warm fresh whole blood transfusion for severe hemorrhage: US military and potential civilian applications. Crit Care Med 2008;36:S340–5.

14. American College of Surgeons Committee on Trauma. Advanced trauma life support program for doctors: ATLS. 6th edition. Chicago (IL): American College of Surgeons; 1997.

15. Cosgriff N, Moore EE, Sauaia A, et al. Predicting life threatening coagulopathy in the massively transfused trauma patient: hypothermia and acidoses revisited. J Trauma 1997;42:857–62.

16. Kermode J, Zheng Q, Milner EP. Marked temperature dependence of the platelet calcium signal induced by human von Willebrand factor. Blood 1999;94:199–207.

17. Morrison CA, Carrick MM, Norman MA, et al. Hypotensive resuscitation strategy reduces transfusion requirements and severe postoperative coagulopathy in trauma patients with hemorrhagic shock: preliminary results of a randomized controlled trial. J Trauma 2011;70:652–63.

18. Mannucci PM, Levi M. Prevention and treatment of major blood loss. N Engl J Med 2007;356:2301–11.

19. Gruen RL, Mitra B. Tranexamic acid for trauma [editorial]. Lancet 2011:1–2.

20. Capan LM, Miller SM. Anesthesia for trauma and burn patients. In: Barash PG, Cullen BF, Stoelting RK, et al, editors. Clinical anesthesia. 6th edition. Philadelphia: Lippincott Williams & Wilkins; 2009. p. 918–9.

21. Romlin B, Petruson K, Nilsson K. Moderate superficial hypothermia prolongs bleeding time in humans. Acta Anaesthesiol Scand 2007;51:198–201.

22. Grant AG. Update on hemostasis: neurosurgery. Surgery 2007;142(Suppl 4):S55–60.

23. Baranov D, Neligan P. Trauma and aggressive homeostasis management. Anesthesiol Clin 2007;25:49–63.

24. Martini W, Pusateri AE, Uscilowicz JM, et al. Independent contributions of hypothermia and acidosis to coagulopathy in swine. J Trauma 2005;58:1002–10.

25. Ireland S, Endacott R, Cameron P, et al. The incidence and significance of accidental hypothermia in major trauma-A prospective observational study. Resuscitation 2011; 82:300–6.

26. Eichhorn JH. Evolution of ASA monitoring standards continues atthe 1998 ASA annual meeting: temperature monitoring controversy. ASA Newsl 1999;63:3.

27. Sessler DI. Temperature monitoring: patterns of intraoperative hypothermia. In: Miller RD, editor. Miller's anesthesia. 6th edition. Orlando: Churchill Livingstone;2005. Chapter 40.

28. Beekley AC. Damage control resuscitation: a sensible approach to the S. exsanguinating surgical patient. Crit Care Med 2008;36:S267–274.

29. Brohi K, Cohen MJ, Davenport RA. Acute coagulopathy of trauma: mechanism, identification and effect. Curr Opin Crit Care 2007;13:680–5.

30. Martini WZ. Trauma associated coagulation disorders: acidosis, hypothermia and coagulopathy. Wien Klin Wochenschr 2010;122(Suppl 5):S4–S5.

31. Engstrom M, Schott U, Nordstrom CH, et al. Increased lactate levels impair the coagulation system: a potential contributing factor to progressive hemorrhage after traumatic brain injury. J Neurosurg Anesthesiol 200;18:200–204.

32. Martini WZ, Dubick MA, Wade CE, Holcomb JB. Evaluation of tris-hydroxyS. methylaminomethane on reversing coagulation abnormalities caused by acidosis in pigs. Crit Care Med 2007;35:1568–74.

33. Koch CG, Li L, Sessler DI, et al. Duration of red-cell storage and complications S. after cardiac surgery. N Engl J Med 2008;358:1229–39.

34. American Society of Anesthesiologists Task Force on Perioperative Blood S. Transfusion and Adjuvant Therapies. Practice guidelines for perioperative blood transfusion and adjuvant therapies. Anesthesiology 2006;105:198–208.

35. Innerhofer P. Dilutional coagulopathy: an underestimated problem? J Anästh Intensivbehandlung 2005;12:212.

36. Levy JH. Massive transfusion coagulopathy. Semin Hematol 2006;43:S59–63.

37. Hoffman M, Monroe DM. Coagulation 2006: a modern view of hemostasis. Hematol Oncol Clin North Am 2007;21:1–11.

38. Fries D, Innerhofer P, Reif C, et al. The effect of fibrinogen substitution on reversal of dilutional coagulopathy: an in vitro model. Anesth Analg 2006;102:347–51.

39. Fukuda T, Nakashima Y, Harada M, et al. Effect of whole blood clotting time in rats with ionized hypocalcemia induced by rapid intravenous citrate infusion. J Toxicol Sci 2006;31:229–34.

40. Hess JR, Lawson JH. The coagulopathy of trauma versus disseminated intravascular coagulation. J Trauma 2006;60:S12–9.

41. Vandromme MJ, Griffin RL, Kerby JD, et al. Identifying risk for massive transfusion in the relatively normotensive patient: utility of the prehospital shock index. J Trauma 2011;70:384–90.

42. Brohi K, Cohen MJ, Ganter MT, et al. Acute traumatic coagulopathy: initiated by hypoperfusion—modulated through the protein C pathway? Ann Surg 2007;245: 812–8.

43. Capan LM, Miller SM. Trauma and burns. In: Barash PG, Cullen BF, Stoelting RK, editors. Clinical anesthesia. 5th edition. Philadelphia: Lippincott Williams & Wilkins; 2006. p. 1262–97.

44. Lier H, Kampe S, Schroder S. Prerequisites of a functional haemostasis. What must be considered at the scene of an accident, in the emergency room and during an operation? Anaesthetist 2007;56:239–51.

45. Kheirabadi BS, Crissey JM, Deguzman R, Holcomb JB. In vivo bleeding time and in vitro thromboelastography measurements are better indicators of dilutional hypothermic coagulopathy than prothrombin time. J Trauma 2007;62:1352–9.

46. Engstrom M, Schott U, Romner B, et al. Acidosis impairs the coagulation: a thromboelastographic study. J Trauma 2006;61:624–8.

47. Holcomb JB, Wade CE, Michalek JE, et al. Increased plasma and platelet to red blood cell ratios improves outcome in 466 massively transfused civilian trauma patients. Ann Surg 2008;248:447–58.

48. Mayer SA, Brun NC, Begtrup K, et al, for the FAST Trial Investigators. Efficacy and safety of recombinant activated factor VII for acute intracerebral hemorrhage. N Engl J Med 2008;358:2127–7.

49. Kashuk JL, Moore EE, Johnson JL, et al. Postinjury life threatening coagulopathy: is 1:1 fresh frozen plasma: packed red blood cells the answer? J Trauma 2008;65:261–71.

50. Shuja F, Finkelstein RA, Fukudome E, et al. Development and testing of low-volume hyperoncotic, hyperosmotic spray-dried plasma for the treatment of trauma-associated coagulopathy. J Trauma 2011;70:664–71.

51. CRASH-2 trial collaborators. The importance of early treatment with tranexamic acid in bleeding trauma patients: an exploratory analysis of CRASH-2 randomised controlled trial. Lancet 2011;377:1096–101.

52. Alam HB, Burris D, DaCorta JA, Rhee P. Hemorrhage control in the battlefield: role of new hemostatic agents. Mil Med 2005;170:63–9.

53. Despotis G, Eby C, Lublin DM. A review of transfusion risks and optimal management of perioperative bleeding with cardiac surgery. Transfusion 2008;48(Suppl 1): 2S–30S.

54. Habler O, Meier J, Pape A, et al. Tolerance to perioperative anemia: mechanisms, influencing factors and limits. Anaesthetist 2006;55:1142–56.

High-Tech, High-Stress Environment: Coping Strategies for the Perioperative Nurse

Vernell Flood, RN, MSN, PMHCNS-BC*, David Allen, MSN, RN, CCRN, CCNS-BC

KEYWORDS

- Coping skills • Perioperative nursing • Stress • Technology

The operating room (OR) is among the most technologically advanced environments within the healthcare profession. This high-tech environment has a unique set of occupational demands that can cause increased stress for the nursing staff. Situations that lead nurses to experience pressure in the OR include the need to work quickly, to face higher medical dispute risks, to work uncertain shifts, to handle precision instruments, and to master complex techniques.[1] Along with this, perioperative nurses are struggling with heavy workloads, high patient acuity, various instrument processing issues, low morale, and staff shortages.[2] The nurse must skillfully manage all of these tasks while keeping patient safety at the fulcrum of it all. Interestingly, the most intense stressor perceived by OR nurses was patient safety.[1] In addition to the occupational stressors that are involved in the OR setting, there are a myriad of interpersonal stressors. The manner in which staff communicate can often times be unprofessional and lead to unresolved conflict and hostile working environments. Recent studies have found that OR nurses felt bullied by other nurses and perceived themselves to be victims of physician-perpetrated abuse.[3,4] Undoubtedly, the culmination of daily stressors that the perioperative nurse encounters can have adverse effects on one's personal and professional life.

Like perioperative nurses, burn nurses at the US Army Institute of Surgical Research experience increased amounts of occupational stress. Nurses in the Burn Center provide care for patients with inhalation injuries, circumferential extremity burns, and general burns of the body. This challenging patient population requires that the nursing staff have the necessary skills to communication with the patient and their families concerning issues such as complex wound care to include pain control along with death and dying. These are sensitive topics that normally elicit emotion

Department of Behavioral Health, United States Army Institute of Surgical Research, 3698 Chambers Pass, Fort Sam Houston, TX 78234-6315, USA

* Corresponding author.

E-mail address: Vernell.flood@us.army.mil

Perioperative Nursing Clinics 7 (2012) 129–133
doi:10.1016/j.cpen.2011.10.004
1556-7931/12/$ – see front matter Published by Elsevier Inc.

response from both the patient and their family members. Imagine the fear of having painful thermal burns covering 20% of your body. Now imagine the excruciating pain involved when the nurse has to scrub the burned skin to clean the affected area. As a result the patient is medicated to help decrease the pain that is experienced during this painful procedure. What about the nurses that are performing these procedures? Do they experience compassion fatigue?

Perioperative and burn nurses would fare better if they could completely eliminate all stress from the workplace. This is impossible, because stress is inevitable whether it be eustress or distress. The key is to limit the impact of occupational stress on the overall quality of life. This can be accomplished by gaining an understanding of the definition of what stress is, identify the negative effects of stress, and learn to implement effective coping skills on a daily basis. Occupational stress is defined as the harmful physical and emotional responses that occur when the requirements of the job do not match the capabilities, resources, or needs of the worker.[5] To gain a better understanding of job stressors, the National Institute for Occupational Stress and Health has developed 6 broad categories that describe the various types of job stressors. They are (1) job or task demands, (2) organizational factors, (3) financial and economic factors, (4) conflict between work and family roles and responsibilities, (5) training and career development issues, and (6) poor organizational climate.[5] All of the stressors that the perioperative nurse experiences can be placed into one of the aforementioned categories.

Regardless of whether the stressors derive from poor interpersonal communications or lack of training on the specialized equipment, the negative mental, emotional, physical, and behavioral impacts that they can have on the perioperative and burn nurse ultimately are the same. Mental symptoms of stress include making careless mistakes, feelings of inadequacy, low self-esteem, and loss of memory. Emotional symptoms include irritability, anger, anxiety, job dissatisfaction, depression, numbness, and feeling drained. Physically, the nurse may feel tired, and experience headaches, changes in blood pressure, muscle tension, or episodes of palpitations. Behaviorally, the person may have insomnia, change eating habits, increase smoking or drinking, isolation, make careless mistakes, not listen to others, pass the buck, have a lack of planning, communicate poorly, experience a lack of sympathy, display a lack of commitment, absenteeism, and power struggles.[5–7] Each person responds to stress differently. It is important to recognize the symptoms of stress as early as possible. Early recognition can prevent eustress from evolving into distress by implementing healthy coping strategies. Optimally, occupational stressors can be managed by making changes at an organizational level.

All parties should be involved and changes improve the working conditions. The most effective way of reducing occupational stressors is to either redesign jobs or make organizational changes.[5] Suggestions of the National Institute for Occupational Stress and Health include ensuring that the workload is in line with the workers' capabilities and resources, clearly defining workers' roles and responsibilities, giving workers opportunities to participate in decisions and actions affecting their jobs, improving communication, reducing uncertainty about career development and future employment prospects, and providing opportunities for social interaction among workers. Often times, organizational change can be a complicated process that requires process improvement and evidence-based project initiatives that include risk/benefit and cost analyses. The nurse may not be the sole decision maker for changes at this level because organizational changes must be approved through multiple layers of leadership.

The perioperative and burn nurse should learn worker-focused stress techniques while awaiting the implementation of organizational level changes. Daily implementation of simple coping strategies will assist the nurse with improving job satisfaction and performance. Just as the flight attendant directs you to apply the oxygen mask to yourself before assisting others in emergency situations during flight, similarly this guidance should apply to the perioperative nurse in performing patient care duties. You must first care for yourself before you can optimally care for others. Listed below are simple strategies to assist in coping with occupational stressors.[5,6]

GET ADEQUATE REST

Most OR cases start as early as 6:00 AM and the last case can be late in the evening. Emergency cases not listed on the OR schedule further prolong the day. Although the number of hours of required sleep varies, most people require 6 to 8 hours of sleep. If you feel refreshed and alert upon awakening, you are most likely achieving adequate rest. If you feel drained, you should consider going to bed earlier so that you can get more rest.

COGNITIVE–BEHAVIORAL TECHNIQUES

Simply put, cognitive–behavioral techniques can be explained by envisioning a triangle in your mind's eye. One leg of the triangle represents your "thoughts," the other leg represents your "feelings," and the third leg represents your "behavior." Each leg of the triangle impacts the other. Likewise, the way you think about an issue will directly affect your feelings, which in turn affects your behavior. When a stressful situation occurs, and it will, ask yourself what you can do to change the situation. If there are things that you can do to change it, then do so. If you cannot change the situation, change your thinking toward the situation. Accept the things that are not within your control to change and explore ways of managing the negative effects that it will have on the way that you feel and the way that you behave.

EXERCISE AND NUTRITION

Regular exercise and healthy eating habits have multiple benefits. Not only do they improve your physical health, but they improve your psychological health. Exercise at least 3 times a week for not less than 20 minutes each iteration. Make exercise fun; you can jog with a friend, join an exercise group, or take a dance fitness class. Maintain a healthy diet by eating well-balanced meals that contain foods from all of the food groups. Also, limit your caffeine and sugar intake. Initially, you may experience a burst of energy from the sugar or caffeine, but later during the day you may feel more tired or sluggish. Caffeine can also have an effect on your sleep pattern.

PEER SUPPORT

Most nurses enjoy the relationships that they make with their patients while caring for them. They enjoy talking to them and getting to know them as they develop a rapport. Perioperative nurses are not afforded this opportunity because their patients are anesthetized for most of the time. Always have at least 1 person with whom you feel comfortable sharing your positive and negative experiences. The OR department increases the quantity and quality of stress relief courses and offer self-esteem–related training programs to assist OR nursing staff to adopt constructive stress coping strategies.[1] Consider starting a peer support group in your organization. The results may improve job satisfaction and impact patient outcome goals. Most organizations have provider resiliency teams that can assist your department with starting a peer support group.

SELF-MEDICATING

The stressful environment, time constraints, and other stressors incumbent of working in the OR could lead to destructive coping patterns. It is not unusual to want to do things that will make you forget about the stressors of work. Pay close attention to the amount of alcohol, nicotine, and other self-medicating substances in which you might be indulging. Seek behavioral health attention if you suspect that you may need assistance.

MEDITATION AND RELAXATION

You will rarely find a perioperative nurse idly sitting at the nurses' station. Instead, the nurse will either be circulating or standing for extended periods of time monitoring patient safety and maintaining equipment accountability. This can be exhausting. Participate in activities that help you to relax. Consider trying yoga, guided imagery, meditation, prayer, Tai Chi, progressive muscle relaxation, or diaphragmatic breathing.

USE ASSERTIVE COMMUNICATION

Communication between staff while in surgery is usually limited and somewhat task-oriented. To decrease the perception of bullying, it is advantageous to communicate with one another in a more effective manner. Use assertive communication instead of passive or aggressive. The assertive communicator is able to disclose thoughts, feelings, and opinions of an event while respecting the rights of others and allowing them to share and provide feedback as well. There will be occasions when the staff will have to agree to disagree on issues in effort to maintain a healthy working environment and relationship. If you would like to gain insight on how you typically respond to conflict in the workplace, consider taking the Thomas–Kilman "Conflict MODE Instrument."[8]

WORK AS A TEAM IN THE OR

Acute stress is increasingly recognized as a factor Implicated in poor OR teamwork.[9] The team found that the circulating nurses are most stressed preoperatively and the assistant surgeons were more stressed intraoperatively and postoperatively. Be mindful of the fact that you and your peers may experience increased stress levels at different junctures of the surgery. Try to be most supportive of one another during these stressful times.

MAINTAIN COMPETENCE

The OR nurses' level of competence was significant for measuring the ability to maintain resilience.[10] The OR is highly technological with new changes and instruments rapidly occurring. Keeping this in mind, it is imperative that the perioperative nurse regularly attends the AORN conference and other training sessions to maintain competency levels. Increased knowledge can decrease stress levels and improve resiliency. The US Army Institute of Surgical Research recognizes the increased need to assist nurses to cope with occupational stressors. According to Melvin,[11] many military healthcare team members have deployed to combat zone at least once in their careers. As a result, they have higher likelihood of being able to identify with their patients, thus having the potential to develop compassion fatigue. To help combat the effects of compassion fatigue, the Institute of Surgical Research established a dedicated psychiatric mental health Clinical Nurse Specialist to provide clinical care to staff members. Furthermore, a tranquility room was developed to help staff members decompress during their shifts. The tranquility room is a dimly lit and has equipment available to help the staff decompress, including an electronic message chair and table. Soothing music is played while the staff member relaxes. The utilization of this service is highly encouraged by management in the Burn Center. The perioperative and burn nurse will experience occupational stress on a daily basis. It is inevitable. Stress mismanagement can affect the perioperative nurse, the patient, and the organization as a whole. On the other hand, managing stress in a healthy way will foster a win–win situation for everyone involved. Eustress will not evolve into distress if you invest time to consistently implement effective coping strategies.

REFERENCES

1. Chen C, Lin C, Wang SL, et al. A study of job stress, stress coping strategies, and job satisfaction for nurses working in middle-level hospital operating rooms. J Nurs Res 2009;17:199–11.
2. Young LE. Mentoring new nursing in stressful times. Can Oper Room Nurs J 2009;27(2):6–30.
3. Vessey JA, Demarco RF, Gaffney DA, et al. Bullying of staff registered nurses in the workplace: a preliminary study for developing personal and organizational strategies for the transformation of hostile to healthy workplace environments. J Prof Nurs 2009;25:299–306.
4. Higgins BL, MacIntosh J. Operating room nurses' perceptions of the effects of physician-perpetrated abuse. Int Nurs Rev 2010;57:321–7.
5. National Institute for Occupational Safety and Health. Exposure to stress: occupational hazards in hospitals. (2008). Available at: www.cdc.gov/niosh. Accessed October 8, 2011.
6. National Health Service. Take control of stress. (2005). Available at: http://www.nhsemployers.org/stress. Accessed October 8, 2011.
7. Hawksley B. Work-related stress, work/life balance and personal life coaching. Br J Commun Nurs 2007;12:34–6.
8. Killman R, Thomas K. Developing a forced-choice measure of conflict-handling behavior: the "MODE" instrument. Educ Psychol Meas 1977;37:309–25.
9. Hull L, Arora S, Kassab E, et al. Assessment of stress and teamwork in the operating room: an exploratory study. Am J Surg 2011;201:24–30.
10. Gillespie B, Chaboyer W, Wallis M, et al. Resilience in the operating room: developing and testing of a resilience model. J Adv Nurs 2007;59:427–38.
11. Serio-Melvin M, Yoder LH, Gaylord KM. Caring for burn patients at the United States Institute of Surgical Research: the nurses' multifaceted roles. Nurs Clin North Am 2010;45(2):233–48.

Behind the Redline: Personal Experiences of a Perioperative Burn Nurse in the Military

Anissa J. Buckley, RN, MSN, CNOR, ACNS

KEYWORDS

- Burn unit • Nursing care • Military nursing
- Perioperative care

In the spring of 2004 I reported to the US Army Institute of Surgical Research (ISR) in San Antonio, Texas, for a 3-year assignment. To be honest I thought, "Why am I going to a research facility if I am a perioperative nurse?" I quickly learned that the ISR has the only Department of Defense burn center in the military. At the time I had been in the military for 7 years and a perioperative nurse for 4 years. Armed with the knowledge of the mission of the ISR and awareness of the conflict occurring in the Middle East, I knew that I was going to work harder than I ever had in my career. Shortly after reporting, I realized that the burn unit was going to have a profound effect on me, not only as a nurse but as a future leader in the US Army Nurse Corps and as a human being. The next 3 years would be a roller coaster of emotions ranging from complete job satisfaction to overwhelming anger.

The burn operating room (OR) is not a typical OR suite. In most operating suites the temperature needs to be in the mid 60s to low 70s to prevent the potential for infection. In the burn OR, the temperature fluctuated from 85° to 100° because the patients were unable to maintain their body temperature due to their burn injuries. The greater the total body surface area (TBSA) burned, the higher the room temperature had to be to compensate for the injury sustained.

When I first reported to the burn OR I was one of two perioperative nurses in one surgical suite. My head nurse at the time, Lieutenant Colonel Pettit-Willis, and I both worked 5 days a week, with our days not ending until all the cases were completed. The 24/7 call schedule was divided among the two of us, averaging 15 days of each month. There were many times when the caseload and/or acuity of the patients

The views expressed herein are the private views of the author and do not necessarily reflect those of the United States Army Institute of Surgical Research, the Army Nurse Corps, the United States Army, or the Department of Defense

McDonald Army Health Center, 576 Jefferson Road, Newport News, VA 23604-5548, USA

E-mail address: Anissa.buckley@us.army.mil

Perioperative Nursing Clinics 7 (2012) 135–138
doi:10.1016/j.cpen.2011.10.002
1556-7931/12/$ – see front matter Published by Elsevier Inc.

became too much for one nurse to handle. When this occurred we cared for the patients together as a team. It was not unusual for us to work 10- to 14-hour shifts straight without relief. With only two nurses circulating in the OR suite, relief usually came only when the cases were completed.

A typical day started between 5:30 AM and 8:00 AM, depending on the number of cases for the day. The days that the flight team brought patients back from Landstuhl, Germany, were always very busy. The patients would arrive in the hospital, get admitted to their wards, and immediately be sent to the OR. The order of surgery was prioritized based on the extent of the patient's injuries. There were days we would have two cases and other days we would have six.

What continually amazed me was how quickly from the point of injury that we had the patient in the OR. A soldier injured in the sands of Iraq could be in the ISR OR in less than 72 hours, a testimony to the collaboration of the services in streaming evacuation care. I firmly believe that the rapid evacuation from point of injury to the ISR made the chances for survival and recovery exponentially greater for the patients treated.

At times I thought it was more difficult for the surgical technicians working in the burn OR. As a circulator, I could walk out of the room for a minute to cool off, but the surgical techs were not as fortunate. Often they would be scrubbed in for many hours and bundled in impervious surgical garb, and I would do my best to keep them focused by supplying them with fluids or hard candy. The ISR maintained a contract for Gatorade drinks, and we would get cases of Gatorade every week. It was important to replace the electrolytes staff lost while in the room. So as busy as the room was on a daily basis, throughout the day I always tried to give the techs bottles of Gatorade or water, using a red robin catheter as a straw.

In early 2004 we had only four surgical technicians and one anesthesiologist. The total number of staff at the time in the OR was seven. For such a small unit we were doing an enormous amount of work. We worked many hours together and became like a small family, bonding through the closeness and intensity of the workload. Over time, more staff was hired to compensate for the ever-increasing surgical caseload of burn casualties.

In the military we are considered soldiers first, and with that comes mandatory training to maintain our deployability and readiness for missions. Ideally we would have up to 12 surgical team members in the OR suite during a surgical case. This team typically included four to five surgical providers, two anesthesia providers, two surgical technicians, one to two circulating nurses, and one respiratory technician. However on days that a military nurse or surgical technician had mandatory training, the team worked short, which negatively impacted the workload and made our day even more challenging.

When I think about the patients that I cared for during my tour in the burn unit there are a few that will stand out in my memory forever. Two in particular come to mind: one was the first patient I cared for in the OR, and the other was a fierce Marine. Both patients had a profound effect on me in different ways.

The very first burn patient I cared for was a young female sailor in her twenties who was involved in a motor vehicle accident while on R & R in Italy. She was flown from Italy to the ISR and taken to surgery within 24 hours of her arrival. She was covered from head to toe in dressings. As we took down the dressings I saw the extent of her injuries and thought, "How is this young girl going to survive?" She was burned over approximately 70% to 75% of her body. As I stood there cutting off the dressing I also thought, "How am I going to be able to look at burned patients every day for 3 years?"

As months went by the amount of her dressings decreased, the number of surgeries decreased, her condition improved, she was transferred from the intensive care unit to the step-down ward, and she regained mobility in her extremities. Then one day as I was walking out of the hospital, I saw a young female sailor walking toward me. I looked at her name tag and realized it was that first burn patient. I said hello as we got closer and stated that I was one of the nurses on duty the day she was brought to the OR. She thanked me for being part of the team that took such great care of her. As I walked away I thought to myself that every minute in the OR with the temperature above 80° was worth it. To see a former patient of mine walking around in her uniform once again was priceless. It was then that I realized I was part of an extraordinary and talented team affording burn patients a fighting chance. Survival was due to the cutting-edge care provided by a highly talented multidisciplinary team.

The fierce Marine, a patient who would have the most lasting impression on me, arrived at the ISR in February 2005. He was a 19-year-old soldier who had sustained a burn of 97% TBSA while on a combat mission as a tank gunner. His job was to spot improvised explosive devices (IEDs) and warn his unit. On the day of his injury he spotted an IED but was unable to warn his unit quickly enough. The first day he was brought to the OR one thought kept going through my mind: "This Marine has the best chance for survival being here at the ISR."

There were about 12 people in the room ready to take care of him. The surgeons decided to harvest the epidermal layer from the 3% of viable skin. The skin was removed with precision using a dermatome, a very sharp surgical instrument for removing very thin layers of skin for use in skin grafting. We took 1-inch diamond-shaped skin samples from his scalp and the soles of his feet. The grafts had to be done with precision to ensure that they could be used as a specimen for future autologous skin grafts. The harvested epidermal skin was sent to a company that grew cultured autologous skin grafts. The process for packing and shipping the skin was just as precise. We read over each step carefully to make sure that everything was done correctly.

Approximately a month later we were notified the autologous epidermal skin was ready for placement. The skin grafts that had been sent to the company were mixed with other cultured skin cells, and the resulting product was called Epicel. The Epicel company representative came to the OR to guide the surgeon in the process of placing the autologous skin grafts. The representative came with multiple small carriers that contained individual trays, each containing one skin graft. The room seemed quieter than usual that day. I believe it was because we all understood the importance each one of the skin grafts had in the survival of the Marine. Each skin graft his body accepted was one less percentage of surface area left to cover.

Placing 1-inch skin grafts on a patient with a 97% TBSA injury was a tedious and precise procedure that took many hours. The whole burn injury could not be completed in one procedure; it required multiple trips to the OR. Each time the Epicel was placed, it was covered with allograft to protect the fragility of the graft. There were days that we opened anywhere from 20 to 50 allografts for the procedure. The Marine was taken to the OR so many times that I lost count of how many procedures he received while in the burn unit.

His total time of admission in the burn unit was 17 months, between the ICU and the step-down ward. He was determined to survive his injuries and be discharged from the hospital. He worked tirelessly in physical therapy to get stronger and to walk again. Every time I saw him during his admission it was apparent that the Marine was one tough kid and that he was not going to give up easily. In December 2006 the hospital had a holiday ball, and the Marine was in attendance. He danced with his mother in front of all of the guests. He proved to everyone that he had survived his burn injuries. There was not a dry eye in the place when they saw him stand up and start slow-dancing with his mother.

In April of 2008 the Marine lost his fight for survival. It had been a little over 3 years that he had survived, and he had started to live his life again. During his rehabilitation he set up a charity for pediatric burn victims. He designed and made T-shirts that he sold to raise money for the pediatric charity. The front of the T-shirt read, "You have a 3% chance of living; what are you going to do?" The back read, "(A) fight through, (B) stay strong, (C) overcome because I am a warrior, (D) all of the above." While in the ISR the fierce Marine fought every day while continuing to be strong, and he overcame his burn injuries. It is only fitting that the letter D was circled on the shirt, because he was a fighter and a warrior. I am honored to say that I own one of his T-shirts, and every time I wear it I remember the fierce Marine.

I mentioned earlier the roller coaster of emotions during my tour. While taking care of the Marine, I definitely had moments of anger. My anger was related to thoughts about the type of people these soldiers were encountering. Sometimes I would catch myself looking at one of the patients and thinking, "How could someone hurt another human in such a traumatic or violent way?" Most of the patients we cared for were less than 30 years of age. In my eyes they were children who had just graduated high school and had not even started to really live their lives. Now they were faced with burn injuries, traumatic injuries, amputations, and the risk of death. When I talked to the patients I would ask if they were angry about what had happened to them. Most of them told me that in the beginning they were angry about their injuries, but later the anger was more about letting their unit down. The unit would now have to fight with one less soldier. Many of the patients spoke of speeding up rehabilitation so they could return to their unit. It was then that I realized my patients did not want my sympathy; they wanted to be respected for what they had done for their country.

There are countless stories about the brave patients the ISR team took care of, both military and civilian. I am incredibly fortunate to have been assigned to a facility that touched and changed so many lives every day, including my own. The knowledge and experience that I gained in 3 years has had a profound effect on my life and career. In the military, personnel are discouraged from returning to a place they were assigned to previously. For me, it would be an honor to serve again at the ISR.

Index

Note: Page numbers of article titles are in **boldface** type.

A

ABCs, of burn resuscitation, 54–56
Acetaminophen, 84
Acidosis, coagulopathy in, 119–120
Acupuncture, 85
Acute lung injury, 16
Acute respiratory distress syndrome, 16
Admission
  to burn center, 35–36
  to burn progressive care unit, 99–100
Airway
  management of, 31
  preoperative evaluation of, 27, 39, 54
Alcohol abuse, in stress, 132
AlloDerm, 6, 48
Allografts, 47, 65–66
American Association of PeriOperative Registered Nurses, pressure ulcer prevention
  guidelines of, 95–96
American Burn Association, National Burn Repository of, 9, 37–38, 93
Analgesia, virtual, 87–88
Anemia, intraoperative, 30
Anesthesia, **23–34**
  burn-related considerations in, 23–24
  for electrical injuries, 31–32
  for excision and grafting, 25–26
  for nonthermal skin diseases, 32
  for out-of-operating room procedures, 31
  for resuscitation phase, 24–25
  for ultrarapid opioid detoxification, **77–81**
  for wound closure, 62
  induction of, 29, 43–44
  inhalational, 30
  intraoperative, 29–31
  monitoring during, 29
  operating setup and, 26
  postanesthesia care for, 20, 31
  preoperative evaluation for, 27–29
  pressure ulcer risk and, 94
  regional, 85–86
Antibiotics, preoperative, 29

Perioperative Nursing Clinics 7 (2012) 139–149
doi:10.1016/S1556-7931(12)00010-1
1556-7931/12/$ – see front matter © 2012 Elsevier Inc. All rights reserved.

periopnursing.theclinics.com

Antimicrobial agents, 25, 50
  history of, 4–5
  in resuscitation phase, 58–59
Anxiety, management of, 67
Assertive communication, for stress management, 132
Autonomic nervous system, response of, 14–15

B

Bacitracin, 5, 50
Battlefield, burn treatment on, **53–69**
  reconstruction phase of, 67
  resuscitation phase of, 54–60
  wound closure phase of, 61–67
Benzodiazepines, 67
Biobrane, 6, 48, 58
Blair knives, 42, 44–45
Blood gas measurement, 30
Blood transfusions. *See* Transfusions.
Bony prominences, pressure ulcer formation at, 89–90
Bovie electrocautery, in wound closure, 63
Braden Scale for Predicting Pressure Sore Risk, 94–95
Bradykinin, release of, 15–16
Breathing, preoperative evaluation of, 39, 54
"Bricks," for massive transfusion, 74–75
Bronchoscopy, for smoke inhalation, 39
Burn(s)
  causes of, 37–38
  characteristics of, 36
  classification of, 12–14, 72–73
  deep partial-thickness, 12–13, 72–73
  depth of, 39
  first-degree (superficial), 12–13, 36, 72–73
  fourth-degree, 14, 36
  in combat, 53
  incidence of, 9, 53
  mortality prediction in, 38
  partial-thickness, 12–13, 72–73
  pathophysiology of, **9–17**
  second-degree (superficial), 12–13, 36, 72–73
  severity of, 38
  statistics on, 37–38
  third-degree (full-thickness), 13–14, 36, 72–73
  types of, 11–12, 72–73
  zones of, 11–12, 38
Burn centers
  admission criteria for, 9–10, 35–36
  specialized, 36–37
  staffing of, 37
  statistics on, 9

Burn progressive care unit, **99–105**
   admission to, 99–100
   discharge from, 103–104
   nutrition support in, 102
   postoperative care in, 103
   routine in, 101–102
   same-day surgery in, 102–103
   transfer to, 100–101
Burn shock, 15–16
   evaluation of, 54
   management of, 92–93
Burn treatment
   anesthesia for. *See* Anesthesia.
   coping strategies for, **129–133**
   history of, **1–8**
   in intensive care unit. *See* Intensive care unit.
   in military. *See* Military.
   multidisciplinary approach to, **77–81**
   nursing experiences with, **135–138**
   pain control in. *See* Pain control.
   perioperative nursing care in, **19–21, 35–52**
   pressure ulcer management in, **89–97**
   progressive care unit for, **99–105**
   reconstructive surgery in. *See* Reconstruction.
   terminology of, 51
   transportation in, 72
   with coagulopathy, **115–127**

   C

"Cadillac of pain control," 85–86
Canaday, skin grafts by, 2
Catecholamines, release of, 15–16
Chlorhexidine, 44, 62
Circulatory system, preoperative evaluation of, 28, 39, 54
Clotting factors, loss of, coagulopathy in, 121
Clysis, hypodermal, 75
Coagulation, zone of, 11
Coagulopathy, trauma-induced, **115–127**
   causes of, 117
   factors affecting, 118–122
   historical perspective of, 116–118
   treatment of, 122–124
Cognitive-behavioral techniques, for stress management, 131
"Combat pill pack," 84
Communication
   assertive, for stress management, 132
   postoperative, 50
Compartment syndrome, versus extremity eschar syndrome, 59
Competence, maintenance of, 132–133
Contractures, surgery for, 102–103

Copeland, dressing techniques of, 6
Coping strategies, **129–133**
CRASH-1 trial, on coagulopathy, 123
Cultured epidermal autograft, 49
Custom-made packs, 41

D

Dakin solution, 4–5, 50
Debridement
   equipment for, 41–42
   in resuscitation phase, 57–58
Decompressive laparotomy, 24–25
Dermacarrier board, 42, 46
Dermatome
   for graft harvesting, 42, 45
   for wound closure, 62
   history of, 4
Dermis, anatomy of, 10
Detoxification, opioid, ultrarapid technique for, **77–81**
Disability, preoperative evaluation of, 55
Discharge, from burn progressive care unit, 103–104
Dobutamine, 74
Donor sites, for grafts, 45–46
   dressing for, 50, 66, 75
   selection of, 110
Dressings, 49
   for burn progressive care unit, 103
   for resuscitation phase, 58–59
   for wound closure, 62, 64–65
   history of, 6–7

E

Eber Papyrus, burn treatment in, 2
Edema, 15–16, 92–93
Edinburgh Royal Infirmary, as first burn hospital, 2
Elderly persons, pressure ulcer risk in, 93
Electric injuries, 31–32
Electrocautery, 39, 63
Environment
   excess heat in, 43, 136
   maintenance of, 55, 61
   stressful nature of, 50–51
Epicel skin substitute, 6
Epidermal autografts, 6
Epidermis, anatomy of, 10
Epinephrine, 43
   for wound closure, 61
   release of, 15–16
Erythema multiforme, 37

Escharotomy, 24–25, 39, 59–60
Excision and grafting, 44–48, 71–75. *See also* Skin grafts.
   equipment for, 41–42
   technique for, 25–26, 62–66
Excisional therapy, 3–4
Exercise, for stress management, 131
Extremities, preoperative evaluation of, 55
Extremity eschar syndrome, 59–60

F

Face, skin grafts for, 66
Fascial excision, 44–45, 63, 73
Fasciotomy, 24–25, 39, 59
Fentanyl, 84
Fibrin sealant, 48
Fibrinolysis, coagulopathy in, 121
Fight or flight response, 14–15
Fire
   prehistoric discovery of, 1–2
   sources of, 37
Flap closures, 112
Fluid therapy, 74–75
   coagulopathy due to, 115–122
   in resuscitation phase, 24–25, 54–55
   in ultrarapid detoxification under anesthesia, 79
   postoperative, 66–67
Fluid warming basin, 42–43
Free-flap closures, 112
Friction, in pressure ulcer formation, 90–91
Full-thickness skin grafts, 46, 109–110

G

Gastrointestinal abnormalities, 16
Girdner, skin grafts by, 3
Goulian knives, 41–42
Grafts, skin. *See* Skin grafts.
Grounding pad, 40–41

H

Hand, skin grafts for, 66
Heat intensity, causing burn, 11
Hemodilution, coagulopathy in, 121
Hemorrhage, in trauma-induced coagulopathy, **115–127**
Hemostasis, 61
   in trauma-induced coagulopathy, **115–127**
   in wound closure, 64
   intraoperative, 30
Hildanus, burn classification by, 2
Histamine, release of, 15–16

Hydromorphone, 67, 84
Hydrosurgical debridement system, 41
Hyperemia, zone of, 11–12
Hypermetabolism, 15–16, 93
Hypodermal clysis, 75
Hypothalamic-pituitary-adrenal axis, response of, 14–15
Hypothermia
  coagulopathy in, 118–119
  prevention of, 40, 74
Hypovolemia, intraoperative, 30

I

Identification band, in operating room, 44
Immersive virtual reality therapy, for pain, 87–88
Immobilization, of skin grafts, 65
Infections, risk factors for, 93
Inflammatory mediators, 15–16
Inhalational anesthesia, 30
Institute of Surgical Research
  burn progressive care unit of, **99–105**
  rule of ten, 55
Integra skin substitute, 5–6, 48
Integumentary system, physiology of, 10
Intensive care unit, **71–75**
  transfer from, to burn progressive care unit, 100–101
  transfer to, from operating room, 50
Intraoperative care
  anesthesia considerations in, 29–31
  in reconstruction, 112
  nurse's role in, 19–21
  pressure ulcer formation during, 90, 94
Intubation, in resuscitation phase, 25

K

Ketamine, 30, 67, 84–85
Kidney dysfunction, 16
Knives, 41–42

L

"Lethal triad of death," 117
Leukotrienes, release of, 15–16
Lidocaine patches, 85
Lorazepam, 67
Lund-Browder burn chart, 55
Lung, complications in, 16

M

Mafenide acetate, 5, 49, 58–59
Mattresses, for pressure ulcer prevention, 95–96

Mechanical ventilation
    anesthesia with, 27
    in ultrarapid detoxification under anesthesia, 79
Meditation, for stress management, 132
MegaDyne MegaSoft electrode pad, 40–41
Meshed skin grafts, 63, 73
Mesher, 4, 42, 46
Metabolic acidosis, coagulopathy in, 119–120
Methadone, 67
Military
    burn statistics in, 38
    burn treatment in
        anesthesia for, **23–34**
        coping strategies for, **129–133**
        history of, 3–4
        nurse's personal experiences in, **135–138**
        on battlefield, **53–69, 83–88**
        pain control in. See Pain control.
        progressive care unit for, **99–105**
        with coagulopathy, **115–127**
Moisture, in pressure ulcer formation, 90–91, 96
Morphine, 84
Mortality, in burns, 38
Multiple organ dysfunction syndrome, risk factors for, 93
Muscle relaxants, 29

N

National Burn Repository
    pressure ulcer data from, 93
    statistics of, 9, 37–38
National Institute for Occupational Stress and Health, job stressors categories of, 130
Negative-pressure wound therapy, 50
Nerve blocks, 85–86
Neurologic system, preoperative evaluation of, 28
Nicotine use, in stress, 132
Nonsteroidal antiinflammatory drugs, 84
Norepinephrine, 15–16, 74
Normothermia, for coagulopathy, 123–124
Nutrition
    for burn progressive care unit, 102
    for stress management, 131
    inadequate, pressure ulcer formation in, 93
    preoperative, 28

O

Obese persons, positioning of, 44
Occlusive dressings, 7
Occupational burns, 37
Occupational stress, coping strategies for, **129–133**
Ollier, skin grafts by, 3
Open exposure method, 6

Operating room
    excess heat in, 43, 136
    patient admission to, 43–44
    preparation of, 40–43
Opioids, detoxification for, ultrarapid technique for, **77–81**
Overlays, for mattresses, 95–96

P

Pain control
    after wound closure, 67
    in battlefield, **83–88**
    in burn progressive care unit, 103
    in wound care, 31
    multidisciplinary approach to, **77–81**
Paraffin treatment, 3
Parkland formula, 55
Pediatric patients
    burns in, causes of, 37
    Parkland formula for, 55
Pedicled closures, 112
Peer support, for stress management, 131–132
Peripheral nerve blocks, 85–86
Petrolatum gauze dressing, 6–7
Picric acid treatment, 3
Pitkin machine, 41
Plastic surgery. *See* Reconstruction.
Positioning
    for excision and grafting, 72
    for pressure ulcer prevention, 94
    for surgical treatment, 43–44
Postanesthesia care unit, 20
Postoperative care, 31
    in burn progressive care unit, 103
    in reconstruction, 112
    in wound closure, 66–67
    nurse's role in, 19–21
Preoperative care
    evaluation in, 27–29, 38–39, 43, 54–56
    in reconstruction, 112
    nurse's role in, 19–21
Pressure ulcers, **89–97**
    economic impact of, 89–90
    formation of, 90–91
    in burn injury, 91–94
    intraoperative considerations with, 94
    prediction of, 94–95
    prevalence of, 89
    prevention of, 89, 95–96
    risk factors for, 90–91, 94–95
    stages of, 90

Propofol, 30
Prostaglandins, release of, 15–16
Pulmonary function, preoperative evaluation of, 27

R

Reconstruction, 67, **107–113**
  in burn progressive care unit, 102–103
  intraoperative care in, 112
  need for, 107
  philosophy of, 107–109
  postoperative care in, 112
  preoperative care in, 112
  techniques for, 109–112
"Reconstructive ladder," 108
Recovery room, 31
Regional anesthesia, 85–86
Relaxation, for stress management, 132
Respiratory failure, in resuscitation phase, 25
Respiratory system, preoperative evaluation of, 27
Respiratory therapy, 72, 79
Rest, for stress management, 131
Resuscitation, 24–25, 38–39, 54–60
  in trauma-induced coagulopathy, **115–127**
  postoperative, 66–67
Reverdin, skin grafts by, 2–3
Rocuronium, 29
Rule of nines, 55
Rule of ten, 55

S

San Antonio Military Medical Center, burn progressive care unit of, **99–105**
Scarring, reconstructive surgery for, 102–103, **107–113**
Self-medicating, in stress, 132
Sepsis, risk factors for, 93
Shear, in pressure ulcer formation, 90–91
Sheet grafts, 45–46, 73–74
Shock, burn. *See* Burn shock.
Silver nitrate, 5, 7, 25, 49
Silver nylon dressings, 64
Silver sulfadiazine, 5, 25, 49, 58–59
Situation-background-assessment-recommendation technique, 50
S-ketamine, 84–85
Skin, physiology of, 10
Skin grafts, 25–26, 45–48
  anesthesia for, 26
  case examples of, 137–138
  for reconstruction, 109–111
  harvesting of, 26, 42, 45–46, 62–63, 110
  history of, 2–4

site preparation for, 62–63
  technique for, 62–66
  tools for, 4
  types of, 45–47
Skin substitutes, 48–49
  history of, 5–6
  in resuscitation phase, 58
SMART team, 99
Smoke inhalation, 39
Sodium hypochlorite, 4–5
Specialty beds, 72
Split-thickness skin grafts, 45, 109–111
Staples, for skin graft fixation, 48, 64
Stasis, zone of, 11
Stevens-Johnson syndrome, 37
Stress, coping strategies for, **129–133**
Stress response, in burn injury, 14–15
Subcutaneous tissue, anatomy of, 10
Susrata, plastic surgery by, 2

T

Tagliacozzi, skin grafts by, 2
Tangential excision, 44, 63–64, 72–73
Tannic acid treatment, 3
Team approach
  for burn treatment, 37
  for stress management, 132
Technology, coping strategies for, **129–133**
Thoracic eschar syndrome, 59–60
Thromboelastography, in coagulopathy, 121–122
Tissue conductance, 11
Tissue tolerance, pressure ulcer formation and, 90
Tools, for wound closure, 61–62
Topical antimicrobial agents, 25, 50
  history of, 4–5
  in resuscitation phase, 58–59
Total body surface area, 37–38
Tourniquets, 41, 61
Toxic epidermal necrolysis syndrome, 32, 36–37
Tracheostomy tube, 27, 50
Tranexamic acid, for coagulopathy, 123
Tranquility room, for stress management, 133
TransCyte, 6, 48
Transdermal analgesia, 84
Transfers
  to burn progressive care unit, 100–101
  to intensive care unit, 50
Transfusions, 30
  "brick" for, 74–75
  coagulopathy due to, 74–75
  postoperative, 67

Transportation, to operating room, 72
Trauma, coagulopathy in. *See* Coagulopathy, trauma-induced.

U

Ulcers, pressure. *See* Pressure ulcers.
Ultrarapid opioid detoxification under anesthesia, **77–81**
United States Army Burn Center, 23–24
    history of, 4
    intensive care unit in, **71–75**
    nurse's personal experience with, **135–138**

V

Vacuum-assisted closure, 50, 64
Vascular access, for surgery, 28
Vasodilatation, pressure ulcer risk and, 94
Vasopressin, 74
Vecuronium, 29
Virtual reality therapy, for pain, 87–88

W

Wallace, dressing techniques of, 6
Watson knives, 42
Weck knives, 41–42, 44–45
Wound care, in resuscitation phase, 56–59
Wound closure
    of special areas, 66
    planning for, 61–62
    postoperative care for, 66–67
    surgical technique for, 62–66
Wound Vacs, 73

X

Xenografts, 47
Xeroform, for graft donor sites, 66

Z

Zimmer dermatome, for wound closure, 62
Zones, of burns, 11–12, 38
Z-plasty, 109

Moving?

Make sure your subscription moves with you!

To notify us of your new address, find your **Clinics Account Number** (located on your mailing label above your name), and contact customer service at:

Email: journalscustomerservice-usa@elsevier.com

800-654-2452 (subscribers in the U.S. & Canada)
314-447-8871 (subscribers outside of the U.S. & Canada)

Fax number: 314-447-8029

Elsevier Health Sciences Division
Subscription Customer Service
3251 Riverport Lane
Maryland Heights, MO 63043

*To ensure uninterrupted delivery of your subscription, please notify us at least 4 weeks in advance of move.

Printed and bound by CPI Group (UK) Ltd, Croydon, CR0 4YY

03/10/2024

01040453-0014